Teaching Patients with Low Literacy Skills

2nd Edition

TEACHING PATIENTS WITH LOW LITERACY SKILLS

2ND EDITION

CECILIA CONRATH DOAK, M.P.H.
DIRECTOR OF EDUCATION
PATIENT LEARNING ASSOCIATES, INC.,
POTOMAC, MD

LEONARD G. DOAK, B.S., P.E.
PRESIDENT
PATIENT LEARNING ASSOCIATES, INC.,
POTOMAC, MD

JANE H. ROOT, Ph.D.
CONSULTANT/TRAINER
HEALTH LITERACY CENTER
UNIVERSITY OF NEW ENGLAND
BIDDEFORD, ME

J. B. Lippincott Company
Philadelphia

Sponsoring Editor: Margaret Belcher
Production Manager: Mary Kinsella
Production/Composition: Berliner, Inc.
Printer/Binder: Courier/Kendallville

Second Edition

6

ISBN 0-397-55161-4

Library of Congress Cataloging-in-Publication Data

Doak, Cecilia Conrath.
    Teaching patients with low literacy skills / Cecilia C. Doak,
Leonard G. Doak, Jane H. Root.—2nd ed.
        p.   cm.
    Includes bibliographical references and index.
    ISBN 0-397-55161-4
    1. Patient education. 2. Socially handicapped—Education.
3. Literacy. I. Doak, Leonard G. II. Root, Jane H. III. Title.
    [DNLM: 1. Patient Education—methods. 2. Educational Status.
3. Teaching Materials.   W 85 D631t 1995]
R727.4.D63 1996
615.5′07—dc20
DNLM/DLC
for Library of Congress   95-11640
                           CIP

♾ This Paper Meets the Requirements of ANSI/NISO Z39.48–1992

Any procedure or practice described in this book should be applied by the health care practitioner under appropriate supervision in accordance with professional standards of care used with regard to the unique circumstances that apply in each practice situation. Care has been taken to confirm the accuracy of information presented and to describe generally accepted practices. However, the authors, editors, and publisher cannot accept any responsibility for errors or omissions or for any consequences from application of the information in this book and make no warranty, express or implied, with respect to the contents of the book.

FOREWORD

Here at last! The second edition of *Teaching Patients with Low Literacy Skills*. Long awaited by many of us–health-care providers and health educators–who have been inspired and instructed by its authors over the years. It is a pleasure to read this book and to reflect on the accumulated wisdom and clear thinking it contains, borne of years of experience and careful listening to the patients we serve.

Marginal literacy was a condition I always had associated with developing countries, not of particular relevance to U.S. health-care providers. This changed for me in 1987. At that time, our agency was working to set up high blood pressure control programs in Philadelphia. We had diagnosed hypertension in 25 percent of our adult population, but 40 percent had dropped out of treatment. *Noncompliant* or *nonadherent* were terms we used for these patients. Searching for ways to promote more effective blood pressure control, I made the rounds of inner-city primary-care practices, speaking to physicians and nurses, offering them stacks of patient information on high blood pressure.

In practice after practice, I received the same message: "No, thank you, I can't use pamphlets; my patients don't read them." At this same time, my colleagues and I were fortunate enough to attend one of the early workshops given by Cecilia and Leonard Doak in Philadelphia in 1987. The workshop demonstrated how most health education messages, including those on high blood pressure control, were not comprehensible to the majority of people whom we were trying to reach. What we subsequently learned about how adults learn, and the nature of the literacy problems, changed our approach to health education forever. We began our own Health Literacy Project in 1988.

Since it was first published in 1985, *Teaching Patients with Low Literacy Skills* has become the major resource book available to health providers who knew that their patients weren't getting the message. The Doaks and Jane Root were the sole voices cautioning health educators to check on not only the medical accuracy of their instructions but the "quality of the learning aspects of the instruction" as well.

Teaching Patients addressed "the mismatch between the literacy skills of Americans and the literacy demands of health-care instruction" and linked principles of health education and adult education. For myself and many of the professionals we have trained, the use of low literacy patient teaching techniques provides a breath of fresh air, empowering to patients and gratifying to us.

Many years have passed. Thousands of copies have been swapped, passed around, and are dog-eared from use. The literature on health and literacy has grown enormously, much of it informed and inspired by the early work of the Doaks and Jane Root. But surprisingly enough, this second edition of *Teaching Patients with Low Literacy Skills* will still be the *only* book on the topic. It, too, pays careful attention to both theory and application and offers us teaching skills that are always respectful of clients, practical, and cost-effective.

It also is attentive to the needs of health professionals. Written directly to the reader, in the personal and user-friendly style that characterizes all their teaching, each chapter gives detailed but clear instructions on how to use various patient teaching techniques and suggests specific activities.

Those readers already familiar with the first edition of *Teaching Patients* will be delighted and intrigued by the second edition. Several features I noted are of immediate use to me. First, a description of the REALM test for assessing clients' literacy skills in the health-care setting is included along with instructions on how to use it. Second is the Doaks' own Suitability Assessment of Materials (SAM) tool, which they recommend using to assess the appropriateness of materials for low literacy populations. A special feature of this tool, which goes far beyond readability, is its suggested method of assessing cultural appropriateness–critical in the United States today.

Third, and breathtaking in its simplicity and clarity, is a new chapter describing health education and adult education theories: what they are, which ones are appropriate for low literacy populations, and why and how to use them in patient teaching. This chapter, like all others, is thoroughly and thoughtfully referenced to expedite further study.

The Appendixes are worth the price of the book. They include the actual REALM test, a summary of the latest data on literacy levels including the 1993 National Adult Literacy Survey, clear and simple instructions on how to lay out an easy-to-read pamphlet, and tips on how to do effective field testing of materials called "Learner Verification and Revision."

Despite the press of time, health professionals at all levels are showing a high degree of learner readiness for information on how to teach growing numbers of patients who are very stressed, very sick, non-English-speaking, poor, and in many cases, come from oral or nonreading cultures.

As now required by JCAHO (Joint Commission on Accreditation of Healthcare Organizations) guidelines, hospitals are taking a look at their consent forms, advance directives, procedure instructions, and a multitude of other patient communications to see if they are understandable and culturally acceptable. Behind this increased interest lies several years worth of national health-care reform debates that have moved the status of disease prevention and its counterpart, patient education, to center stage.

For those who strive to build effective patient education–health professionals, health-care administrators, faculty and students in the health-care professions–this book will be extraordinarily useful. Happy reading!

Sarah B. Furnas, R.N.
Director, Professional Services
Health Promotion Council of Southeastern Pennsylvania
Philadelphia, PA

PREFACE

The second edition of *Teaching Patients with Low Literacy Skills* comes from the combined experiences of three authors who share a common concern for patients who have difficulty understanding health-care instructions due to their limited literacy skills. All three have had years of experience as volunteer tutors of adult nonreaders. Over the past ten years, the authors have conducted more than 200 workshops to train nurses, doctors, and other health-care practitioners in methods to make health-care instructions easier to understand.

Len and Ceci Doak (a husband and wife team) have analyzed more than 2,000 health-care instructions in all media, and provided advice on changes to make them more user-friendly for patients. Dr. Jane Root, with her colleagues at the Maine Area Health Education Center, has developed and patient tested scores of easy-to-read health materials. The results of these experiences, together with recent research, and the findings from a number of health education projects have been brought together in this second edition.

The second edition is intended for health-care practitioners and those who teach them. The new edition provides ideas, methods, and examples on how to simplify health instructions so that they are understood better by patients at all literacy levels—including those with low literacy skills.

Two new chapters have been included in this edition: Chapter 2, Applying Theory in Practice, and Chapter 8, Teaching with Technology. Chapter 2 provides guidance on applying behavior and learning theories in the design of health-care instructions. Chapter 8 offers practical advice and examples on teaching with audiotapes, videotapes, and multimedia—all of which are growing rapidly for patient education. As much as possible, each chapter has been made a complete unit of information on its subject, and provides extensive references.

The reader who is faced with the task of developing a written instruction will find that Chapter 6, Writing the Message, offers guidance and examples on both the planning and development steps. If visuals are to be included with the written message, Chapter 7, Visuals and How to Use Them, offers guidelines and examples.

We have tried to make our suggestions practical and useful to busy health practitioners who have little extra time. Since the research shows that well-educated adults learn much more from simply written material than from more difficult material, this edition has been written at an easy-to-read 7th- to 11th-grade level.

Health education is an inherent part of the practice of virtually all nurses, doctors, and other health practitioners. Health maintenance requires patient understanding of instructions, and is becoming an increasing role for all in the health-care field. The Joint Commission on the Accreditation of Health Organizations (JCAHO) has recognized this by elevating the importance of patient comprehension of health instructions in the accreditation process. All patients (or their guardians) can learn almost anything they need to know for their health care if it is taught appropriately. This second edition is dedicated to the health-care practitioners who are striving to achieve that goal.

Cecilia Conrath Doak, M.P.H.
Leonard G. Doak, P.E.
Jane S. Root, Ph.D.

ACKNOWLEDGMENTS

We express our deepest thanks to the reviewers of our manuscript, all of whom are authorities in their specialities. Their careful reflections on what we wrote sharpened our perceptions and helped to keep us focused on our objective. Their lively discussion of the content often changed our ideas, sometimes challenged our concepts, and always improved the outcome. Our conviction in the benefits of learner verification and revision is stronger than ever! The reviewers are to be commended for their excellent comments.

The reviewers of the entire manuscript are:

GWEN COLLINS, RN, BSN
Patient Educator, Staff Educator, Nurse Supervisor
HCA Palmyra Medical Center
Albany, Georgia

DOROTHY GOHDES, MD
Director, Diabetes Control Program
Indian Health Service
Albuquerque, New Mexico

JEANNETTE SIMMONS, DSc
Clinical Professor (retired)
Department of Community and Family Medicine
Dartmouth Medical School
Hanover, New Hampshire

The reviewers of special chapters are:

GODFREY HOCHBAUM, PhD
Professor of Health Education (retired)
School of Public Health
University of North Carolina
Chapel Hill, North Carolina

MARJORIE SCHARF, MPH, RD
Nutrition Consultant
Philadelphia Department of Public Health
Philadelphia, Pennsylvania

JANET WEINER, RD, MS, LD
Metro Health Maternity and Infant Care Program
Cleveland, Ohio

RALPH WILEMAN, PhD
Professor, School of Education
University of North Carolina
Chapel Hill, North Carolina

CONTENTS

1

"Where are all the people who can't read? We don't see them in our practice."

The Literacy Problem

A typical scenario in hospitals and clinics across the United States:

DOCTOR: Do you understand what to do when you get home?
PATIENT: Oh, yes.
DOCTOR: Well, here's a pamphlet with all the facts. Read this if you have any questions.

The doctor's comments sound reasonable enough, but literacy authorities tell us that 27 million American adults—nearly one out of five—may not be able to read a pamphlet. A recent survey by the National Center for Educational Statistics shows that 40 to 44 million adults have literacy competency skills at the lowest level. They can understand only the simplest written instructions.[1]

Limitations of Low Literacy Patients

Those with low literacy skills can't read pamphlets or booklets, directions on a bottle of aspirin, or the explanations for a food exchange list. Vocabulary is not their only limitation; often they can't understand the illustrations and medical pictures used in health-care materials.

They have no visible signs of literacy disability—you cannot identify them by appearance or casual conversation. They may be poor or affluent, native born or immigrant, and they are found everywhere. Health care providers treat them by the tens of thousands every day.

1

The good news is that the great majority of this population is deficient only in literacy skills—not in intelligence. They can learn from nearly any health instruction that is designed and presented in ways suitable for them. Unhappily, a great many health care instructions fall far short of being suitable and thus are not understood and accepted by patients.

The purpose of this book is to provide ideas, information, guidelines, and examples that will help you design and present health messages suitable for all segments of the public—your patient population.

This chapter addresses the mismatch between the literacy skills of Americans and the literacy demands of their health care instructions. Subsequent chapters deal with how health care providers can cope with the literacy mismatch. This chapter discusses:

- The magnitude of the literacy problem and what it means to you
- Differences between skilled and unskilled readers and the impact on health care
- Myths about literacy
- Research and trends to reduce the impact of illiteracy on health care

Who Is Literate?

Until a few years ago, literacy skills were universally measured in terms of **grade level**—the average reading skill achieved at each year of schooling in the American public school system. Readability levels of texts were also rated by school grade level. A person who can read at the 5th-grade level or higher was considered literate. Those who read at less than 5th-grade level are sometimes referred to as functionally illiterate.

More recently, an alternative method of defining literacy skills came into use: **functional competency levels.** This method measures the ability of people to perform literacy tasks over a range of difficulty levels. People are said to be functionally competent (in literacy) when their literacy skills permit them to fully function in society. Functional competency is assessed by means of a multi-task literacy test, the results of which are scored on a scale of 0 to 500.

For ease of understanding, the numerical data (0 to 500) from literacy surveys are also reported in five groups or levels. Level 1 is the lowest and level 5 is the highest. Functional competency measures are used in literacy surveys sponsored by government agencies.

These two literacy measures, grade level and functional competency, use different measurement criteria and there is no direct conversion between them. However, as a rough approximation, one may say that those who read below 5th-grade level correspond with those whose literacy skills fall in level 1 in terms of functional competency in literacy tasks.

Regardless of which literacy definition is used, state and national surveys indicate that a large number of adult Americans, roughly one out of five, have serious literacy limitations.

The Magnitude of the Literacy Problem

In summary, the following statements describe a literacy cross section of adult Americans—a cross section of the average adult patient population:

- The *average* reading level is at the 8th- to 9th-grade level (between levels 2 and 3 in functional competency measures).
- About *one out of five* read at the 5th-grade level and below (in functional competency terms, at about level 1).
- For older Americans (65 and over) and for inner-city minorities almost *two out of five* read below the 5th-grade level (at level 1).

Figure 1-1 shows, in graphic format, the profiles of the literacy skills of Americans. Additional data from national literacy surveys are given in Appendix A.

What do these charts mean? They tell us that the lowest group—about 20 percent of adult Americans—is functionally illiterate. They can't read most newspapers (these are at 9th- to 12th-grade readability levels) or directions on a box of cake mix. The charts also tell us that another group—about 30 percent—has *marginal* reading skills. Most written health care instructions available today are at readability levels that are "over the heads" of both groups.

Impact of Literacy Skills on Health Care

Like all people, those with low literacy skills get sick, go to doctors and clinics, sometimes are hospitalized, and most of all, like the rest of us, they want to recover as quickly as possible. The challenge faced by health practitioners

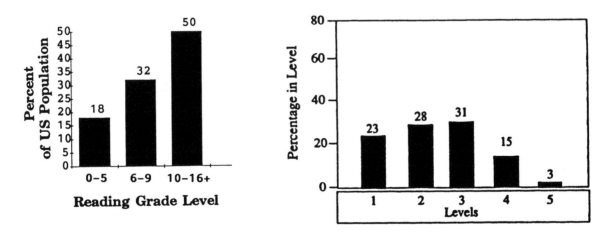

FIGURE 1-1

Reading skills of adult Americans by **grade levels** *(left graph)* and **functional competency** *(right graph)*

is how to cope with a large patient population that does not have well-developed skills in reading, writing, listening, or speaking. The task is to work around the literacy barriers so that these patients can carry out at least a critical minimum set of instructions to manage their health care.

Low literacy has an impact on the cost of health care. Weiss et al. (1993) found that those with the lowest literacy skills required far greater medical care than those with even marginal literacy skills.[2] People with low literacy skills seem to put off disease prevention actions and to wait longer before seeking medical help. The former point was reinforced by the health officer for Washington, DC, who reported that parents with the lowest literacy skills are far more likely to ignore written notices to bring their infants to a clinic for immunizations.

Differences Between Skilled and Poor Readers

Poor readers obtain much less from health care instructions than do skilled readers. This is true even for materials that have fairly low readability levels.[3] Poor readers may read most or all of the words in an instruction and still obtain little or no meaning from the text. The reasons for this are outlined in Table 1-1, along with strategies that health practitioners can use to manage these literacy problems.

Poor readers take instructions literally without interpreting them differently for new situations.

Treatment and health care management may be unfamiliar subjects to many patients. Without a broader context or an explanation of the limitations or circumstances, a patient may follow the instruction to the letter, even when it makes no sense. For example, in order for the patient to examine her stools over the following weeks for a black color that might indicate intestinal bleeding, the doctor told the patient not to eat beets. The patient never ate beets again for the remaining 15 years of her life. A more tragic example told by a physician is as follows:

A baby was brought to the clinic with diarrhea. I treated the baby and told the mother to "push fluids" with the baby. That was about 8 A.M. The mother brought the baby home, and at noon the baby was dead. The mother had literally pushed fluids by tipping the baby's bottle upside-down and forcing the fluid when the baby's responses began to slow down. The baby suffocated.[4]

TABLE 1-1

Differences between good and poor readers—and how you can manage the problems

SKILLED READERS	POOR READERS	MANAGING THE PROBLEMS
Interpret meaning	Take words literally	Explain the meaning
Read with fluency	Read slowly, miss meaning	Use common words, examples
Get help for uncommon word	Skip over the word	Use examples, review
Grasp the context	Miss the context	Tell context first, use visuals
Persistent reader	Tire quickly	Short segments, easy layout

To the patient who is motivated to follow instructions, the literal meaning may be the only message that comes across.

Poor readers often read (decode) one word at a time.

When people read one word at a time they often forget the preceding words by the time they get to the end of the sentence. Thus, the text they've read provides no meaning. Anderson et al. (1985) observe that "poor readers read at a rate so slow as to interfere with comprehension even of easy materials."[5]

For example, it is not difficult to imagine that the instruction, "Alcoholic ingestion superimposed upon inadequate dietary intake can precipitate acute hyperglycemia," will make little sense to many readers—even those with good reading skills. A simpler instruction might say: "Don't drink alcohol on an empty stomach. It can cause hyperglycemia." But even simple sentences, with just one or two uncommon words, can have the same slowing-down effect on poor readers.

Poor readers don't think in terms of classes of information or categories, and they skip over uncommon words.

Patients may think in terms of the individual items rather than a class of information; they may not know the meaning of category words used in health care instructions.

For example, many cannot use the yellow pages of the telephone book because they do not understand the category words used in the listings. The grouping of foods into the four food groups or classes is also difficult for many. Even common category words may not be understood. After reading a paragraph that said to eat red meat and to avoid shellfish and poultry, one patient on dialysis mentioned that he eats lots of fried chicken. When asked, "What about poultry?" he replied, "Oh, I never eat poultry. We're not supposed to have that!"

Poor readers may miss the context and not make inferences from factual data.

Poor readers may not make inferences as to changes in their own behaviors that are *implied* in displays of statistical information or disease etiology.

For example, the patient cited in the exchange with the doctor at the beginning of this chapter may not perceive that the factual data in the pamphlet (what happened to other people) have any connection with his own life unless this is explained.

In summary, although many people with low literacy skills have adequate intelligence, they tend to have less well-developed skills in reading, and in analysis and synthesis.

Common Myths About Literacy/Illiteracy

MYTH: *"Illiterates are dumb and learn slowly, if at all."* — *FALSE*

> Throughout the world almost 800 million people are illiterate, mainly due to economic reasons rather than because of low intelligence. Most people with low literacy skills have average IQs and function quite well by compensating in other ways for the lack of reading skills.

MYTH: *"Most illiterates are poor, immigrants, or minorities."* — *FALSE*

> In terms of the U.S. population, most are white native-born Americans, and are found in every walk of life. On a percentage basis, more minorities and immigrants do have reading difficulties.

MYTH: *"People will tell you if they can't read."* — *FALSE*

> Since there is a strong social stigma attached to illiteracy, nearly all nonreaders or poor readers will seek to conceal this fact. They will use ruses such as, "I forgot my glasses," or, "I'll have to take this home for my husband (wife) to see it first," or, "My eyes are tired." Consequences can be serious if medication directions are not followed, or merely inconvenient for the patient who could not read a sign.

> I had to go to the clinic for x-rays. The girl at the desk told me which room to go to and I went in and sat down. Quite a few people came in. Pretty soon I saw that those who came after me were called, but I never was. I sat there for nearly an hour before I asked the nurse when my turn was. She asked if I had signed the register. When I said, "No," she pointed to the sign at the front of her desk and she read, "Please sign the register when you come in." I didn't tell her I couldn't read. She took me next. (personal communication from Literacy Volunteers of America Inc., 1980)

MYTH: *"Years of schooling is a good measure of literacy level."* — *FALSE*

> Years of schooling tells what people have been exposed to, not what reading skill they acquired. Surveys have shown that, on average, adults currently read three to five grade levels lower than the years of schooling completed.[6] Through disuse, the reading skills of many adults have atrophied.

Trends in Health Education That Address Low Literacy Issues

> Over the past several years there has been a broad societal movement toward simpler text. The movement is seen in the Plain Language Laws passed by many state legislatures. Simplified directives have also been promulgated at

the federal level. President Carter signed Executive Order 12044 to mandate the use of plain language in all government departments.

Do good readers feel "talked down to" by simply written health materials? On the contrary, people at all literacy levels can better understand and indeed have a preference for simpler rather than more complex written materials.[7]

Throughout American industry, literacy and skills training programs are now common.[8] As a part of these programs, extensive effort is also going into task analysis inherent in work elements and the assessment of literacy skills required to perform each task. These task analysis methods could also be applied by health practitioners to assess the literacy demand of tasks assigned to patients.

The health community has also taken action. Since 1993, the Joint Commission of Accreditation of Health Organizations (JCAHO) has included in the accreditation scoring how well patients *understand* their health care instructions. Health organizations are now scored on how well their patients understand:

- The safe and effective use of medication
- The safe and effective use of medical equipment
- Potential food–drug interactions
- When and how to obtain further treatment

Additional factors have been added to the above JCAHO standards for 1994 and 1995.

Federal agencies have been active in meeting the health needs of low literacy clients. In 1992 the U.S. Public Health Service funded several million dollars in grants to study ways to more effectively communicate with and motivate those with low literacy skills. The National Cancer Institute, Office of Cancer Communication, has established a National Work Group on Cancer and Literacy. The Centers for Disease Control has issued a reference work on literacy and health and a resource book on effective nonprint health instructions.[9,10]

The Agency for Health Care Policy and Research is developing an extensive series of health care instructions for the public at easy-to-read levels. The Indian Health Service has developed a series of seven easy-to-read (3rd- to 5th-grade levels) diabetes prevention and treatment booklets for Native Americans (Figure 1-2).

Research on methods to cope with the literacy problem in a health context is increasing rapidly. The frequency of this topic at conference sessions, workshops, and technical paper presentations is testimony to its broad interest.

Some health care organizations have established working relationships with national literacy organizations. One cancer information center has developed easy-to-read cancer prevention materials that can be used as adult texts for those studying reading in Adult Basic Education (ABE) classes.[11] The Area Health Education Center (AHEC) in Maine enlists literacy educators as co-authors of new health care materials and has arranged for ABE class participants to pretest the draft health care materials for comprehension.[12]

To reach poor readers, nonprint media are increasingly being used. Rap-song audiotapes on breast self-examination, immunization, nutrition, and

FIGURE 1-2

Easy-to-read diabetes booklets. (*Source:* Indian Health Service)

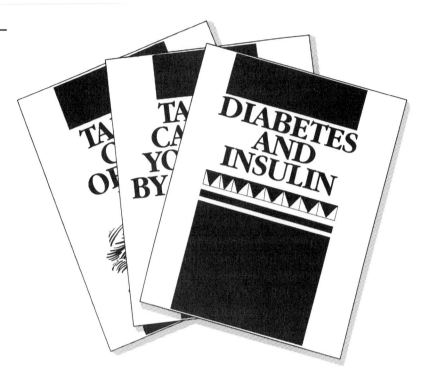

other topics have been developed during the past few years.[13,14] Videos are now available to communicate AIDS (acquired immune deficiency syndrome) prevention via a story line, provide prenatal nutrition instruction to pregnant teenagers, and teach cooking to reduce fat.[15,16,17]

Much is being done and progress is being made. A long-term goal of the U.S. educational system is to raise the country's literacy skills. Until this goal is achieved, the health care community must make health instructions easier to understand. This book is about simplifying health care instructions in practical ways that are within the limits of our time and other resources.

Summary

Literacy skills of Americans range from the nonreader to the highly literate. Half the U.S. population read at the 9th-grade level or lower. Most current health care instructions are above that level.

Those with the lowest literacy skills will understand few written health care materials. For those with the lowest literacy skills alternative (nonprint) formats may be better understood, including audiotapes, simple sketches to show desired behaviors, videotapes, and games. Low reading levels are more common among those over 65 and among inner-city populations of all ages. The key information about the low literacy populations may be summarized as follows:

- About one out of five adult Americans read below the 5th-grade level.
- They do not look to print materials for health information.

- They try to hide their literacy deficiency and usually succeed in doing so.
- Their IQs are adequate. They can learn anything needed for their health care if it is appropriately taught.

The nation's health organizations are increasingly aware of the impact of literacy on health care and health costs. Many have undertaken initiatives to increase awareness of the problem and to improve comprehension of patient instructions. In the chapters that follow, methods are presented that can help make health care instructions easier to understand for all patients.

References

1. Kirsch IS, Jungeblut A, Jenkins L, Kolstad A (September 1993): Adult Literacy in America. National Center for Education Statistics, U.S. Department of Education, Wash., D.C., p. xiv.
2. Weiss BD, Blanchard JS, McGee DL, et al. (1993): Illiteracy Among Medicaid Recipients. Relationship to Health Care Costs. University of Arizona, College of Medicine Report.
3. David TC, Bocchini JA, Fredrickson D, et al. (Fall 1994): Polio vaccine information pamphlets. Study of parent comprehension comparing a short polio vaccine information pamphlet containing graphics and simple language with the currently available Public Health Service brochure. Pediatrics (in press).
4. McKeever N, Conrath C, Skinner ML (1956): Stimulating improved health behavior of American Indians. U.S. Public Health Service. Unpublished.
5. Anderson RC, Heibert AH, Scott JA, Wilkinson IA (1985): Becoming a Nation of Readers. National Institute of Education, U.S. Department of Education.
6. Doak LG, Doak CC (1980): Patient comprehension profiles. Recent findings and strategies. Patient Counseling and Health Education 2(3):101–106.
7. Ley P, Jain VK, Skilbeck CE (1976): A method for decreasing patients' medication errors. Psychological Medicine 6:599–691.
8. Conrath J (July/August 1993): Training: basic skills and quality. Illinois Manufacturer. Illinois Manufacturers Association, Chicago, pp. 11–12.
9. Centers for Disease Control (March 1991): Literacy and Health in the United States. Selected Annotations. CDC, Atlanta.
10. Centers for Disease Control (December 1994): Beyond the Brochure. Alternative Approaches to Health Communication. CDC, Atlanta.
11. Massey Cancer Center, MCV Station Box 37, Richmond, VA 23298-0037. Attn: Dr. Thomas J. Smith.
12. AHEC at the University of New England Literacy Center, 11 Hills Beach Road, Biddeford, ME 04005.
13. Ehmann J (1991): BSE Rap (tape and video), 199 New Scotland Avenue, Albany, NY 12208.
14. Senah C (1991): Zap Goes the Measles (30-second audiotape). Health Education Department, Port of Spain, Trinidad.
15. Women's Council, American Friends Society (1991): Si met ko (videotape on AIDS). New York.
16. Scharf M (1992): Healthy Foods, Healthy Baby (video, poster, booklet), Department of Health, 500 South Broad Street, Philadelphia, PA 19146.
17. Furnas S (1990): Put Away the Frying Pan (10-minute video). Health Promotion Council of Southeast Pennsylvania, Philadelphia, PA 19107.

2

"We have so little time. How can theory help?"

Applying Theory in Practice

Introduction

Theories are a generalized set of rules, and Hochbaum (1992) tells us "they become instruments to search for answers" for patient learning and motivation.[1] They help us predict the consequences of a health education intervention and can save the practitioner from "learning the hard way" that a planned intervention is likely to turn out badly. The need for useful theory has been with us for a long time. Nyswander (1956) says, "For it is in new situations that a good theory is needed by any and all of us.[2]

Theories can provide you with a workable basis for an education action you wish to undertake. This is especially important when teaching low literacy clients whose educational needs may be less predictable. For health educators, the advantages of theories are:

1. They provide a predictable framework to plan education interventions that are more likely to succeed.
2. They offer a means to explain and justify the intervention to colleagues.
3. They give us a blueprint to replicate successful educational interventions.
4. They offer a systematic process to analyze success or failure.

We recognize that practitioners are often too busy to consider the dozens of learning and behavior theories before planning an education intervention. An alternative is suggested. Since there is interrelation and overlap between most theories and models, one need consider only a handful of theories on an everyday basis. In this chapter, we have selected, summarized, and interpreted the most relevant theories to teach patients with low literacy skills. The reader is advised that such summarization has limitations and must omit many details. The full texts on these behavior and learning theories are listed in the References.

The theory and guidelines provide a framework for both teaching and the development of health education materials that are covered in the chapters that follow. This chapter is in two parts. Part 1 deals with theory and how it can be applied; Part 2 translates theory into practice via a set of practical guidelines.

In **Part 1,** we seek to show how theory can help us solve health education problems and answer such practical questions as:

- Which theories should I consider applying during the planning and development of a new or revised health care instruction? How could these theories apply to health education interventions for low literacy clients?
- How do I go about applying these theories?
- How will theory help me deal with instructions for another culture?
- How do the theories apply to clients who have low literacy skills?

In **Part 2,** we present practical guidelines from the theories in Part 1. The guidelines are a "shorthand" way to apply the theories to a wide range of common health education questions. Typical of these are:

- How much can I expect most clients to be able to cope with in one session?
- How much should I include about the medical concepts; the medical vocabulary? What is the best sequence for these topics?
- How can I determine that my patients understand their instructions?
- What must I include in the instruction so it will build a feeling of self-efficacy and acceptance by my clients so they are more likely to comply?

Part 1: The Role of Theory

As with any set of rules, theories should not be followed blindly. Theories are validated under research conditions where nearly all of the variables are held constant. For this reason, one must be careful in applying theories when different variables are operative or when they are used with a different population, situation, or problem than the one originally studied. You must be the judge of how well a given theory applies to your task, situation, and patient population; or whether the theory applies at all. This chapter provides you with advice to help you make that judgment.

Theory you can use

A summary of the theories that are likely to be most useful to you and where they apply are presented in Table 2-1. The table can serve as a quick checklist when you are developing a new health education intervention. In the pages following this table, each theory and its applications are discussed.

TABLE 2-1

A summary of key education and behavior theories and their applications

THEORY NAME	PROPONENTS	DESCRIPTION	APPLICATION
Health Belief Model	Hochbaum Becker Rosenstock Greene	Explains people's health behaviors: why they may accept preventive health services or adopt healthy behaviors.	A behavior research tool, but can imply best content and topic sequence for educ. mat'ls.
Self-Efficacy	Bandura Adams Beyer	People are more likely to adopt a health behavior if they think they can do it.	Intervention should give people confidence by building up to behavior step by step. Give them many little "successes" in the behavior change process.
Locus of Control Theory	Wollston	People who believe *they* are in control of their own health status are more likely to change behaviors in response to health ed. facts. The converse is also true.	For people who believe they are *not* in control, build more support into health ed. programs.
Cognitive Dissonance Theory	Festinger Lewin	A high level of unhappiness (dissonance) is more likely to lead to behavior change. Theory points to readiness to change, and how to cut probability of relapse.	Design intervention to foster unhappiness with present behavior status. To reduce relapse, reinforce to keep dissonance low.
Diffusion Theory	Rogers Shoemaker Preston	Some people will adopt new behaviors early, some late. Early adopters can influence others. Applies to a community or population.	Foster early adoption by making intervention consistent with beliefs, values, social system of target population.
Stages of Readiness	Prochaska	A person goes thru stages of readiness to adopt and to maintain a new health behavior. Ed. interventions work best if they match a person's stage of readiness.	Design intervention to fit the stages of readiness of your client population. If many stages are present, the intervention may need several different messages.
Adult Ed. Theories	Bruner Bradford Coleman Knowles	Main concern of adults is solving & managing their own problems. They care about self-fulfillment. Adults need active participation. Adults are less interested in facts about health as a *subject*.	1) Design ed. intervention to address the solution to their health problem. Give less info about other topics. 2) Build on adult's experience. 3) "Talk it out", teach via demos., discussion and examples.

The Health Belief Model

Description: The Health Belief Model (HBM) tells us that as a general rule, people will respond best to messages on health promotion or disease prevention when they perceive that they are susceptible (at risk), that the risk is serious, that they will receive benefits from a behavior change, and that the barriers to behavior change are not too great.[3–6] The authors believe that to change behaviors, health education interventions are likely to be more effective when the intervention addresses these perceptions. Thus, a logical construct for health education interventions for behavior change is to include the topics shown in Box 2-1.

HBM does *not* tell us that for behavior change we must include such topics as the Greek or Latin derivation of the name of the disease; a description of the disease process; or the national statistics on morbidity or mortality. Unfortunately many of today's health instructions do include these topics.

Exceptions to the content and sequence of information shown in Box 2-1 would include detailed procedures and administrative instructions. Often, for safety or legal reasons, other topics must also be included, such as side effects of medication, and where to go for services. If necessary, consider including such topics *after* the HMB sequence.

Application: The HBM applies where we want to understand what is needed for the patient to make a behavior change. It applies to individuals and groups of people. The HBM offers insights as to the content and sequence of topics in health instructions and, by implication, what not to include.

Health care providers tend to have empathy for their clients and do not like to do anything to raise their anxiety. Janis and Feshbach (1953) tell us that we may need to raise the clients' anxiety (via the "I'm at risk") in order to obtain a certain behavior change.[7] "It is knowing the threat and knowing the concrete ways to cope with it that provide lasting action."[8]

How does the application of the HBM-derived topics in Box 2-1 benefit patients with low literacy skills?

- They provide motivation to change.
- They focus on behavior—"what I can do about it"—so that people know what to do to reduce the risk of anxiety.
- Because simple vocabulary and context can be used to describe behaviors, information about behavior is easier to understand than information about disease processes, physiology, and statistics.

When behavior change is the focus of the education intervention, you can often eliminate complex topics that may be expressed in lists, graphs, charts, and drawings whose formats may be unfamiliar to patients.

BOX 2-1

Content and sequence of topics for health behavior change

- I perceive that I am personally at risk, and the risk is serious.
- I see a way to reduce my risk, and I believe I will benefit if I do it.
- The barriers (pain, cost, etc,) are not too high for me to do it.

Self-Efficacy Theory (the "doability" factor)

Description: The theory addresses the role of people's confidence that they could carry out the behavior asked of them. A person with low self-efficacy is less likely to try to carry out a new health care behavior, or to change an ingrained behavior. Using this theory, the education intervention should build clients' self-confidence that they can do the behavior asked of them. Indeed, Bandura and Adams (1982) suggest that the most important precondition for behavior change is self-efficacy.[9] Rosenstock and others have revised and expanded the HBM to include it.[10]

Factors that help build a patient's self-efficacy are:

- The patient's initial perception or experience is that the task is doable.
- The task, especially a complex task or behavior, is partitioned into smaller, easier-to-do subtasks. This allows many small successes to be experienced during the learning process.
- There is repetition of the task or behavior.
- There is recognition, reward, and reinforcement for doing the task.

Application: Except possibly for the initial client perception of doability, the factors listed above are under the control of the health care provider. You can build these factors into your educational interventions, and often this can be done quite easily.

Initial perception or self-confidence that patients can do a task (or change a behavior) is influenced by the way the topic is introduced and presented. This may be a deciding factor in whether or not clients will pay attention and try to learn from the education intervention. For example, to increase clients' perception of doability, you could begin by mentioning the similarity of the task to something they can already do, by explaining that the task can be done one step at a time, and then citing testimonials from other patients who have done it.

To build self-efficacy, the first step is to partition a complex task (or concept) into subtasks that appear easy to the client. The second step is to offer feedback (reinforcement) to the client after each step.

From the client's viewpoint, what is a complex task or concept? That depends on the client's knowledge, skills, and experience. For example, for many literate people, taking and understanding their own blood pressure is complex. Consider the blood pressure instruction in Table 2-2: the original, and a rewritten version with the same concept divided into two parts. In the rewritten version, note also that interaction has been added. In Part 2 of this chapter, we will say more about the benefits of interaction.

Repetitions build self-confidence and skill—and hence, self-efficacy. Some examples to build self-confidence are: practicing insulin injections; clients showing the dietitian how they can select several low-sodium foods from a list; demonstrating a rehabilitation exercise.

TABLE 2-2
Blood pressure instruction

ORIGINAL	REWRITTEN
WHAT DO THE NUMBERS MEAN? When a health professional takes your blood pressure, it is reported in two numbers such as 120/80. The first number is called the systolic pressure and represents the pressure against the artery walls when the heart beats. The second number, the diastolic pressure, represents the pressure against the artery walls when the heart is resting between beats.	**WHAT DO THE NUMBERS MEAN?** When your blood pressure is taken, you get two numbers—like 120/80. The *first number* is your blood pressure when your heart beats to push your blood. This is the larger number. What is your pressure when your heart beats? Write it here_____. The *second number* is your blood pressure between beats. This is the smaller number. What is your blood pressure between heart beats? Write it here_____. Now you have both numbers: _____ over _____.

Recognition, reward, or reinforcement for the accomplishment of subtasks can build self-esteem and self-confidence. This is especially important for clients who have low literacy skills because during their lives they have often guessed wrong, and hence are more likely to have low self-confidence that they can perform the tasks asked of them. A sincere "Good, you're beginning to get the idea!" or "You've got it right!" from a health care provider, or even a positive response from a computer-aided instruction, can help immensely.

Locus of Control Theory

Description: The theory addresses the impact of how much control people believe they have over their own health. Those who believe or feel that their health is in the hands of God/fate or the doctors (external control) are less inclined to take preventive health actions. The converse is also true: those who feel that they are in charge of their health condition (internal control) are likely to adopt healthy behaviors.

This theory is especially significant for some cultures, and for those who have low literacy skills. The latter, in the past, seldom understood health care instructions. Thus, they feel that managing their own health is beyond their understanding. But external locus of control is not restricted to those with low literacy skills. Even people with high literacy skills may "assign" external locus of control to others in health matters. For example, a college-educated person declined to participate in the agency's wellness program and gave his reason as, "Wellness is not my responsibility; that's my doctor's job. He's supposed to keep me healthy."

Application: How does the health care provider know the locus of control for a given patient? Upon initial contact with a new client, you usually can't tell. People with external locus of control may be difficult to motivate to adopt new health behaviors. The safest course to take in designing or presenting a health education intervention is to frame your message in terms of what actions to take (and that they are doable) rather than in terms of "It's your responsibility to take action."

Cognitive Dissonance Theory

Description: This theory is useful for education interventions to get a person to the point of making a decision and to maintain the behavior once it has been decided. Festinger (1962) defines cognitive dissonance as information or behavior that doesn't fit or is at odds with our overall knowledge, behaviors, or decisions.[11] In other words, we don't feel good when we keep doing things that we know are bad for us. For example, a person who is painfully aware that smoking is unhealthy and wants to quit would likely suffer some cognitive dissonance (mental discomfort) upon realizing he was opening a third pack of cigarettes for the day.

The more important the knowledge, behavior, or decision is to a person, the greater the potential cognitive dissonance. *The theory says that when these pressures are experienced, people seek ways to reduce them.* These pressures may be either positive or negative in terms of health behaviors. In the example cited above, the person might seek to temporarily reduce the cognitive dissonance by promising himself that he will quit smoking tomorrow. The tenets of this theory are summarized in the statements below.

Cognitive Dissonance Theory (CDT)

- People try to reduce the cognitive dissonance in their lives.
- The greater the dissonance, the greater the pressure to make a change that will reduce it. But there is often resistance to doing this. One type of resistance is the freezing effect to stick by our original decisions.
- After patients have made a good decision, reinforcement is needed to keep them from regressing. Reinforcement may take the form of additional supporting information, role models, and addressing environmental factors.
- Changes in behavior lead to changes in attitude to conform to the behavior.

Application: The theory follows the common-sense notion that people prefer to be comfortable in their minds, and when there is discomfort they try to reduce it. Two applications of CDT might be (1) by deliberately increasing patient discomfort about an undesirable behavior, health educators may cause a behavior change, and (2) after the patient has made the desired behavior change, multiple reinforcements of the decision are needed to maintain it.

An increase in mental conflict might arise from peer group pressure to revert to the old, unhealthy behavior. When that happens, reinforcements can serve to lower the mental conflict. A good example of how this can be done is shown in a video instruction on eating right for pregnant teenagers. One sequence shows a peer pressure situation where a pregnant teenager is urged to eat junk food. The video shows a way to respond to that peer pressure and also to build self-esteem by selecting healthy food alternatives.[12]

Diffusion Theory

Description: Diffusion theory deals with the ways that new ideas are communicated (diffused) and adopted throughout a community or a population. The theory recognizes that information paths may be centralized (top down from an authority figure) or diffused (horizontally from a series of peers). Rogers and Shoemaker (1971) tell us that regardless of how the information is communicated, we should not expect everyone to accept a new health behavior recommendation at the same time.[13]

The first people to adopt a new idea are those who are secure enough to feel comfortable in making a change. They tend to be innovators. They may serve as models or "change agents" for others who follow. The next group is the early adopters. Both groups tend to make decisions based on rational thinking and expectancies. To convince the innovators and early adopters to change a health behavior, your message needs to be logical and must present the rationale and proof of results.

Other people will adopt much later. Those who are last to do so, the "late adopters," are likely to be more conservative, impoverished, or less secure. They are moved to adopt more by social influences (local organizations, friends, models) than by rational thinking. For late adopters, health information heard at a neighborhood party is likely to have more influence than advice from a health expert seen on television.[14]

Application: Diffusion theory can help health educators to set more realistic goals and time frames for their programs. The health educator can speed up the process of diffusion (adoption) of a health behavior by initially targeting the health message to the innovators and early adopters in the community. These may be political figures, teachers, successful businesspeople, the socially prominent, or sports stars. The message should include a rational description of health risks, the rationale for change, and the benefits. The health belief model is a suitable format.

Later, when early adopters have made the desired behavior changes, the message may be revised to (1) stress the social influences for the desired behaviors, and (2) target the local community organizations including peer role models.

Stages of Readiness Theory

Description: Prochaska and DiClemente (1985) tell us that a person goes through stages in adopting a new belief or behavior.[15] Thus, the health education intervention should address the needs at the current stage of readiness. These stages are defined as:

1. **Precontemplative:** not aware or not considering a change

2. **Contemplative:** thinking about change, but not taking action
3. **Action:** has made behavior change and is practicing it
4. **Maintenance:** retaining the behavior via reinforcement or learning
5. **Termination:** the end of intervention; the behavior is a part of life and is no longer seen as a change that needs attention or reinforcement

Application: The content of your health message must be geared to the patient's present state of readiness. Your objective is to move the client along to the next stage—perhaps from the contemplative stage to the action stage. For example, it would not be surprising that most newly diagnosed diabetics are likely to be ready to take action to control their condition, so the health messages need to deal with knowledge and skill building to enable them to do so. In many cases, the patient's stage of readiness will not be so obvious.

One way to find out where the patients are in terms of readiness is to set up a small focus group of patients to elicit from them how they view the "problem," their current behavior toward the problem, and what they see as actions that could be taken. (See Chapter 10 for discussion of focus groups.)

People with low literacy skills are less likely than others to obtain health information from written materials. If they are not aware of a health problem (such as the importance of immunization for infants) they are likely to be in the precontemplative stage, and the health education intervention should include awareness topics.

Sometimes the instruction must be suitable for clients at several stages of readiness. In such cases, the instruction must include topics suitable for each of these stages. If you are designing a new instruction (pamphlet, audiotape, videotape, or verbal instruction), decide on the readiness stages of your target audience, and include the content they require.

Adult education

Description: In keeping with the summary nature of this chapter, we will narrow the field of education theory to give emphasis to those theories and research findings dealing with adults with low literacy skills. Having said that, it is important to note that nearly all education methods that work well for those with low literacy skills also work well for those with higher literacy skills.

Characteristics of adult learners

Adults have a large base of life experiences to build upon. They generally know what they want from an educational experience. Cheatham (1993) points out that those with low literacy skills approach education with apprehension.[16] In the past, they have had many failures at learning—sometimes to their embarrassment. The health educator must design the instruction to reduce this apprehension. For instance, an easy-to-use audiotape or computer-aided instruction may be helpful. Research in adult education identifies the characteristics of the adult learner:[17-20]

How we learn

Derryberry and Skinner (1954) suggest we consider the learning conditions in terms of the following factors:[21]

MOTIVATION AND INTEREST

Learning takes place due to motivation within the person, not an outside force. Thus, no matter how clever we are at teaching, our efforts are likely to fail unless the person wants to learn. The patient in a clinic may want to learn because he believes he has a health problem.

This point was further elaborated upon by Roberts (1956), who states that, "The interplay between what people know and how anxious they feel about it determine what action they take. People without the anxiety phenomenon are more likely to delay taking any action."[22] (And that includes learning.)

LEARNING METHODS AND EXPECTATIONS

Learning is an active process. It is a result of our own efforts to learn. So long as a patient is passive about learning, he will learn little. Thus, teaching methods need to include ways to gain attention and must actively involve the patient. Being told what to do, or being given a pamphlet, does not meet this requirement.

INTERPRETATION AND EVALUATION

We interpret new information based on our past experience. What is learned and how it is learned differs from one person to another. Each comes to a learning situation with his or her own unique set of backgrounds and points of view.

People will change behavior only when they understand what to do and can see that taking the action to change behavior furthers achievement of their goals. In health terms, it means knowing what action to take and how it relates to solving their health problem or reducing their health anxiety.

The attitudes of the groups to which the patient belongs are a significant force. Most people tend to conform to the accepted standards and sanctions of family and friends. These may determine whether information is accepted and learned and whether a person takes action.

These characteristics affect both the content and teaching methods of adults and lead to the following suggestions for teaching. (See other tips on teaching in Chapter 9.)

1. *Tell patients that the instruction is aimed at solving/managing their health problem.* Ask about what they know, and then outline the topics you are going to cover in the instruction.
2. *Get to the point quickly.* Patients with low literacy skills tend to have short attention spans and lose interest rapidly. Present the information in the context of benefits in their lives—not in the medical context. Contrast the following statements that illustrate these two contexts: "If you take these

pills every day, you will feel better and you can stay on your job," rather than "I'll give you a prescription for a new medication we're having good clinical results with."

3. *Ask patients to solve a problem with the new information:* ask them to tell or show you how they will use the information just learned. Listen and offer words of encouragement. For example, after instruction but prior to hospital discharge you might ask the patient, "You'll be changing your dressings at home now. If your wife asks you how you will do that, how will you explain to her what you have to do?"

These three suggestions are consistent with the proverbial teaching dictum: "Tell me and I'll forget. Show me and I may remember. Let me do it and I'll learn."

Part 1 has provided an overview of learning and behavior theory as applied to adult patients—including those with low literacy skills. Lewin said that, "There is nothing so practical as a good principle or theory." How can you use these theories on a day-to-day basis?

Steps in applying theory

- When you initiate a new health care instruction, review the theories in Table 2-1.
- Which theories apply to what you're about to do? To your objective; to your client population; to their situation; to their environment?
- What do the theories tell you to consider?

We ask you to stop at this point and take a few minutes to apply the three actions above to the last health instruction you developed or presented. Referring to the theories in Table 2-1, which would apply to your instruction? What do these theories tell you to do to improve the effectiveness of this instruction the next time?

Part 2: Applying Theory to Practice

The initiative to develop a new health care instruction may come from a variety of sources. At the grassroots level, you may do so in response to a new procedure or to a lack of understanding or knowledge on the part of patients. At the national level, legislation has required that standardized health instructions be developed and made available nationwide.[23]

To assure the medical quality of new health care instructions, it is standard procedure for the medical accuracy to be carefully checked. The quality of the learning aspects of the instruction must receive the same careful attention. To move a step closer to that objective, in Part 2 we present a set of guidelines for health instruction materials and teaching that will lead to an increase in their educational quality.

Guidelines for health instructions

The guidelines apply to any instructional media: print, audio, visual, demonstrations. These guidelines can be used with both individual and group instructions. It is not surprising that a common set of guidelines apply to all media because the human brain processes information and stores (learns) it according to a structured set of rules. This chapter deals with those key learning rules that should be built into almost any health education material to make it simple and understandable.

Over the past several years one can observe a broad societal movement toward simpler text. The federal government as well as 25 states have passed legislation toward this end. The legal profession as well has begun to recognize the need for plain English.[24] A frequently asked question is, "But won't people with high literacy skills feel talked down to by instructions that are simple?" There is evidence that people at all knowledge and literacy levels prefer and better understand materials that are simple.[25,26]

One must make a distinction between literature and written information. Health instructions fall in the latter category. Literature can be complex and is often enhanced by allusions, metaphors, and other devices that invite linguistic exploration. The intended outcome is satisfaction and joy. Informational reading, on the other hand, is intended to inform or empower. The language and visuals need to be clear and simple, and the text well organized. This is a formula for health instructions that will be understood by many. Box 2-2 presents guidelines for development of health instruction materials for patients who have low literacy skills.

BOX 2-2

Guidelines for health education methods and materials

1. **SET REALISTIC OBJECTIVE(S)**

   — Limit the objective to what the majority of the target population needs now.
   — Use a planning sheet to write down the objective and key points.

2. **TO CHANGE HEALTH BEHAVIORS, FOCUS ON BEHAVIORS AND SKILLS**

   — Emphasize behaviors and skills rather than facts.
   — Consider the sequence for the topics shown in Box 2-1. Otherwise, consider placing the key points first and last.

3. **PRESENT CONTEXT FIRST (BEFORE GIVING NEW INFORMATION)**

   — State the purpose or use for new content information before presenting it.
   — Relate new information to the context of patients' lives.

4. **PARTITION COMPLEX INSTRUCTIONS**

   — Break instruction into easy-to-understand parts.
   — Provide opportunities for small successes.

5. **MAKE IT INTERACTIVE**

   — Consider including an interaction after each key topic. The patient must: write, tell, show, demonstrate, select, or solve a problem.

Limit the objectives to one or two for most instructions intended for patients and for the general public. If additional objectives are necessary, consider scheduling a separate session or using an additional instructional material.

The objectives should state exactly what actions or behaviors you want to see from the education intervention. To develop an instruction that makes the objective relevant for patients, objectives should be expressed in terms of the *patients' objective* (i.e., translate an objective to lower blood pressure to: "to help you to live to see your grandkids grow up").

It is important to keep the *education objective(s)* separate from other objectives. Otherwise, one may assign objectives to the education intervention that education cannot achieve. The patient may "fail" to comply with the education actions because noneducation objectives or conditions are not met. For instance, an education intervention may have convinced a woman to have a mammogram, but she may fail to do so for environmental, cultural, or economic reasons.

To change behaviors, focus the content on behaviors rather than on facts or principles. Facts and principles may imply what a patient's behavior should be, but low literacy patients may not see the implication. Rely on your objective(s) to decide what outcomes are desired for the patients. Then focus the instruction's content on the behaviors that will lead to these outcomes.

Patients do not need to learn the underlying principles to understand and carry out the behaviors.[27,28,29] This has an important impact on the content of your instructions. To obtain the patient behavior outcomes you seek, you rarely have to include the complex underlying physiological reasons for those behaviors. Thus, your instruction can be both easier to prepare and more understandable by your patient population.

Present the context first—i.e., the framework or purpose of the new information. The context is the part the patient already knows.[30] All of us understand better when we are given the framework or context first, and then the new information. When writing a paragraph, consider making the first sentence or first clause tell where/how the information fits or is to be applied. (For example, in the previous sentence, the first four words, "When writing a paragraph," provide the context for what is to come afterward in the sentence. You know what a paragraph is, so you have a mental framework to contain the information that follows these words.)

For instance, rather than writing, "Broccoli, carrots, sweet potatoes, peas, spinach, cabbage, beets, and squash have many nutrients," it is better to say, "Vegetables with many nutrients are broccoli, carrots, etc. In the former sentence the readers/listeners must try to carry the whole list in memory as individual items with no framework as to how they fit together until they arrive at the end of the sentence. By that time they may have forgotten most or all of the items. On the surface this may seem like a trivial grammatical transposition, but the research shows that it can make a huge difference in patient comprehension and recall.

Partition complex instructions. Think of ways to divide your instruction into a number of small, logical pieces. Procedures and health care lists that exceed seven items are unlikely to be remembered regardless of a person's education or skill level.[31] Such procedures require partitioning or "chunking." For most people three to five items per chunk may be a reasonable limit.

As a way to remember a series of steps in a complex task, consider an easy-to-remember mnemonic. For example, it is easy to remember the three steps in cardiopulmonary resuscitation (CPR) by the instructional mnemonic "A,B,C": Airway, Breathing, Compressions.

Make instructions interactive—i.e., the patient must do, write, say, or show something in response to the instruction. This greatly increases interest in and recall of information, and should be a standard feature in the design of nearly all instructions.[32,33] Medical science has shown that interaction causes a protein change in the brain that stimulates information retention for long-term memory.[34] (See also Chapter 5, The Comprehension Process.)

Effective interactions can be incorporated into health care instructions in any medium. A recent series of 24 nutrition materials (using print, visuals, or video) developed by expert panels for the National Cancer Institute included reader/viewer interactions in each material.[35] When these materials were field tested with sample populations, respondents said they enjoyed, learned, and were motivated by the interactions.[36] Methods to incorporate interaction into text are described in Chapter 6.

For video instructions, interaction should be designed into the programming so that the questions or situations used to obtain interaction follow the information sequence naturally and permit sufficient time for the viewer to interact. A worksheet or checksheet can provide the viewer with a supplemental means to interact with the video. If the instructional videos that you are using do not have interaction built in, you can add it by preparing a worksheet to be used by the patients who view the video. Additional means of interaction are presented in Chapters 7 and 8.

Summary

The five guidelines (Box 2-2) offer a framework for the design of health instructions in any medium. If you use these guidelines in the design and development of your instructions, your patients will more likely understand and accept them. Chapters 6, 7, and 8 show examples in a variety of media that apply the guidelines.

References

1. Hochbaum, GM (Fall 1992): Theory in health education practice. Health Education Quarterly 19(3):296.
2. Nyswander DB (November 1, 1956): Education for health—some principles and their application. California's Health 14(9).
3. Becker MH (1974): The health belief model and personal health behavior. Health Education Monographs 2:324–472.
4. Glanz K, Lewis FM, Rimer B (eds) (1991): Health Behavior and Health Education. Theory, Research and Practice. Chapter 3 by Rosenstock I, The health belief model: explaining behavior through expectancies. San Francisco: Jossey Bass.

5. Becker MH, et al (1977): The health belief model and prediction of dietary compliance: a field experiment. J of Health and Soc Behav 18:348–366.
6. Hochbaum GM (1958): Public Participation in Medical Screening Programs: A Sociopsychological Study. Public Health Services Pub. No. 572.
7. Janis IL, Feshbach S (1953): Effects of fear arousing communications. J Abnorm Soc Psych 48:78.
8. Haynes RB (October 1980): Patient Compliance to Prescribed Antihypertensive Medications: A Report to NHLBI. NIH Pub. 81-2102, pp 22–23.
9. Bandura A, Adams NE (1982): Analysis of self efficacy theory in behavior change. Cognitive Therapy and Research 1:287–310.
10. Rosenstock IM, Strecher VJ, Becker MH (Summer 1988): Social learning theory and the health belief model. Health Education Quarterly 15(2):175–183.
11. Festinger L (1962): A Theory of Cognitive Dissonance. Stanford University Press, Stanford, CA.
12. Scharf M (1992): Healthy Foods, Healthy Baby. Video, 12 minutes, Department of Public Health, Office of Maternal and Infant Health, Philadelphia, PA.
13. Rogers EM, Shoemaker FF (1971): Communication of Innovations, 2nd ed. New York: The Free Press.
14. Robbins K (May 1988): Master of Science thesis. Adaptation of educational reading materials for WIC participants of Dubuque, Iowa. Cardinal Stritch College.
15. Prochaska JO, DiClemente CC (1985): Common process of self change in smoking, weight control, and psychological distress. In Coping and Substance Abuse. New York: Academic Press, pp 345–363.
16. Cheatham JB (1993): TUTOR: A Collaborative Approach to Literacy Instruction. Syracuse, NY: Literacy Volunteers of America Inc., p 22, 1993.
17. Knowles MS (1970): The Modern Practice of Adult Education. New York: Association Press.
18. Knowles MS (1973): The Adult Learner: A Neglected Species, 2nd ed. Houston: Gulf Publishing Company, pp 60–98.
19. Bruner JS (1966): Toward a Theory of Instruction. The Belknap Press of Harvard University. Cambridge, MA.
20. Gage NL (1963): Handbook of Research on Teaching. Chicago: Rand McNally & Co.
21. Derryberry M, Skinner ML (November 1954): Health Education for Outpatients. Public Health Reports, 69, 11:1107–1114. As contained in Derryberry M (1987): Educating for Health: Selected Papers of Mayhew Derryberry. NCHE Press Division of the National Center for Health Education, pp 79–90.
22. Roberts BJ (1956): A study of selected factors and their association with action for medical care (breast cancer). Doctoral dissertation, doctorate of Public Health in Health Education. Harvard University, Boston, MA.
23. Public Law P.L.101-239 (December 1989): Established the Agency for Health Care Policy and Research to provide standardized clinical and patient guidelines to enhance quality appropriateness.
24. Cooley, TM (1992): Law review. Plain English: A charter for clear writing. Michigan Bar Journal 9(1).
25. Ley P, Jain VK, Skilbeck CE (1976): A method for decreasing patients' medication errors. Psychological Medicine 6:599–691.
26. Plimpton S, Root J (January–February 1994): Materials and strategies that work in low literacy health communication. Public Health Reports 109(1):86–92.
27. Bradshaw P, Ley P, Kinsey J (1975): Recall of medical advice: comprehensibility and specificity. Br J Soc Clin Psychol 14:55–62.
28. Rogers M, Shoemaker FE (1971): Communication of Innovations: A Cross Cultural Approach, 2nd ed. New York: The Free Press, pp. 106–107.
29. Knowles MS (1970): The Modern Practice of Adult Education. New York: Association Press.
30. Gopen GD, Swan JA (November–December 1990): The science of scientific writing. American Scientist 78:550–558.
31. Miller GA (1956): The magical number seven. Psychol Rev 63:81.

32. Knowles M (1973): The Adult Learner: A Neglected Species, 2nd ed. Houston: Gulf Publishing Company. See Theories of teaching, pp. 60–98.

33. Gage NL (1963): Handbook of Research on Teaching. Chicago: Rand McNally, pp. 1121–1122.

34. Jonassen DH (ed) (1982): The Technology of Text. Englewood Cliffs, NJ: Educational Technical Publishing Company, pp. 92–93.

35. National Cancer Institute, Office of Cancer Communications (1992): Nutrition Materials for Seven Ethnic Populations That Apply the Nutritional Guidelines for Cancer Prevention.

36. Doak L, Doak C (July/August 1992): Reports to NCI: Ethnic and Low Literacy Nutrition Education Project: Learner Verification Assessment Reports.

3

"How can I test our clients' literacy skills and not embarrass them?"

Testing Literacy Skills of Patients

Testing patients' ability to read and to comprehend written health care instructions is becoming more widespread. Health care providers realize that this information can help them to be more effective in teaching their patients. Knowing your patients' levels of literacy skill and comprehension helps you to:

1. Match the readability level of materials to the reading skills of patients
2. Know whether supplemental teaching is needed when using health care material
3. Know when it is necessary to employ nonprint media such as visuals, demonstration, audiotapes, and videotapes
4. Verify that patients understand their instructions in accordance with the new directives from the Joint Commission on Accreditation of Health Organizations (JCAHO)

This chapter describes several tests that directly measure patient literacy skills. Most of the tests were developed in the field of education and have been in use for many years. Learning to use these testing methods takes very little time: the word recognition tests can be learned in less than an hour, and testing a patient takes no more than 5 minutes. The authors and others who have used these test methods have found that most patients enjoy the attention they receive during the test and they participate willingly.

Additional Rationale for Testing Patients' Literacy Skills

Nurses, doctors, and other health professionals have high literacy skills compared to the population as a whole and therefore they may overestimate the literacy skills of their patients. The assumption is often made that adult patients can read at levels equal to the level of schooling they have completed. This assumption is not supported by literacy surveys, which show that, among the general public, literacy skills are much lower—on the average, about five grade levels lower than the last school year completed.[1] A possible explanation for this gap is that since reading is a skill it atrophies with disuse, as do most other learned skills.

Since years of schooling is not a reliable indicator for literacy skills, why not just ask patients if they read well? Unfortunately, this question is not likely to be productive. In the National Adult Literacy Survey, over two-thirds of those who tested at the very lowest reading level reported that they "read well" or "read very well."[2]

Your purpose in testing a patient population may be (1) to obtain a *profile* of the reading skills (collectively) of your patient population, or (2) to determine the reading skills of *individual* patients. In most cases the testing methods will be the same; only the end uses of the data are different.

A profile of your patient population is useful in planning new or revised education programs. The profile can point to the average readability level needed for instructional materials for your patient population.

On the other hand, testing every patient can help you select the best method to teach an individual patient. You can find out whether an individual has sufficient skill to read instruction materials given to him or her.

Methods to Measure Patient Reading and Comprehension Skills

The ability to read material does not guarantee that the material is understood. Reading and understanding call on different skills. A patient may be able to read all the words in a sentence but not understand its meaning.

Two methods to test patients' reading skills and two methods to test their comprehension are presented in this chapter (see Box 3-1). The *reading skill tests* deal with the ability to decode the words. Decoding is the process of transforming the letters into words and being able to pronounce them correctly. This is an essential step in reading. The *comprehension tests* deals with how much the patient understands from reading.

BOX 3-1

Reading and comprehension tests

I. Reading skill tests
   1. Wide range achievement test (WRAT)
   2. Rapid Estimate of Adult Literacy in Medicine (REALM)

II. Comprehension skill tests
   1. Reading comprehension: Cloze test
   2. Listening comprehension test

In addition to the methods shown in Box 3-1, there are indirect ways to obtain an approximate assessment of patient literacy skills. One approach is to ask your patient to read a short passage from a readability graded health instruction—no more than a page or two. Then ask the patient a few detailed questions about the content of the passage. If the patient can respond correctly to the questions, you can assume that he or she can read text at least at the grade level of the instruction used.

Why not test patients for functional competency in reading with the methods used in the National Adult Literacy Survey (NALS)?[3] We do not recommend this method because the combined test time for prose and document testing of 40 minutes is likely to be too long for most health care settings. A further problem with the use of NALS methods in a health care setting is pointed out in Appendix A.

Part 1: Measuring Reading Skills

The reading process

The reading process is complex. It involves a merging of both language and thinking skills with what we commonly think of as reading. Oral language is the base for reading. To read, we must make the shift from speech to print using a process called *decoding.* The position of decoding in the reading process is shown in Figure 3-1. Decoding is the skill that is measured by the WRAT and the REALM tests mentioned earlier.

Literal comprehension is a step beyond decoding the words—it means that we understand what we read. The Cloze test and the listening test measure comprehension. Another good way to measure whether or not comprehension has taken place is to ask the patient to transform what was read into other words or other formats. That is, to tell you in his own words what the text means, or to demonstrate the procedure described in the text.

FIGURE 3-1

Levels in the reading process. (*Source: Tutor,* Literacy Volunteers of America Inc., Syracuse, NY, 1972, p. 49)

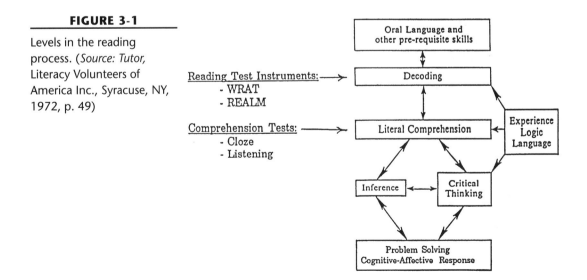

As shown in Figure 3-1, making inferences and problem solving are steps beyond decoding (reading) and literal comprehension. As noted in Chapter 1, many readers with low literacy skills take words literally, and do not draw inferences from written information and data.

Selecting a test method

The **reading skill tests** (part I of Box 3-1) may be used to:

1. Provide a profile of the reading skills of a patient population
2. Provide a reading skill level of individual patients so that teaching materials and methods appropriate to their skill levels are used
3. Serve as a screening threshold for further tests such as the Cloze or to select patients able to read and respond to a questionnaire
4. Provide literacy data for health education research purposes

Although either the WRAT or the REALM could be applied to the four purposes stated above, the REALM may be the most convenient for the first two, and the WRAT more appropriate for the last two because of its higher precision. Since both WRAT and REALM call for reading word lists aloud, the tests must be conducted on an individual rather than a group basis.

Administering the tests: the importance of the introduction

The authors have conducted reading tests with patients in hospital waiting rooms, at bedside, and in the cafeteria. Others have successfully tested people at community centers and on the street.[4] The willingness of people to undergo these tests, and the way they feel after taking them, depend on how they are introduced. Patients are almost always willing to participate if you explain the purpose of the test and ask for their help. It is best to be honest about the purpose. You may start with a statement such as:

"We want to make our instructions easy to understand, so I need to find out how well you can read. To do this I need your help to read some words. It will only take a few minutes. Will you help me?"

The key phrase in the above introduction is "Will you help me?" After the patient agrees, explain briefly what you want her to do, show her the test sheet, and proceed with the test.

Occasionally patients may be confused or reluctant to take the test. For these few it is best not to proceed, but to withdraw the test graciously. Instead, you may consider using the indirect test method mentioned earlier in this chapter. Do not be dismayed if you can't conduct a reading test on every patient. Once in a while, you may find a patient who, for any of a variety of reasons, does not want to be tested at that time.

The WRAT 3 Test (Wide-Range Achievement Test)

The WRAT[5] has been widely normalized with thousands of subjects and has been used to test reading skills in school systems throughout the United States for over 40 years. The current version, WRAT 3, was copyrighted in 1993, and costs about US$99 for a package containing an administration manual, test cards, and scoring sheets. In this test patients read aloud from a list of words of progressive difficulty. The more words they can pronounce correctly, the higher their reading skill.

Many studies that first identified the gap between readability levels of health care materials and reading skills of patients were done by testing patients using the *Reading* portion of the WRAT.[6,7,8] (Other portions of WRAT address writing and numeracy skills.)

To administer the WRAT 3 reading test, explain the purpose of the test as illustrated above. Then present the patient with the card containing the list of words (see Figure 3-2). The patient is asked to read each word aloud, starting with the easiest word on the list of 42 words. The tester listens carefully, following along on a separate word list, and making a check mark over each word that is pronounced incorrectly until 10 consecutive words are mispronounced. Then the test is stopped, the patient is thanked and may be dismissed, and the test is scored.

The *WRAT 3 Manual* provides a reference for correct pronunciation; however, regional and ethnic accent differences are allowed. The *WRAT 3 Administration Manual* is used to convert the number of words pronounced correctly during the test to a reading grade-level score for the patient tested.

FIGURE 3-2

WRAT 3 reading test, partial word list. (© Wide Range Inc., Wilmington, Delaware)

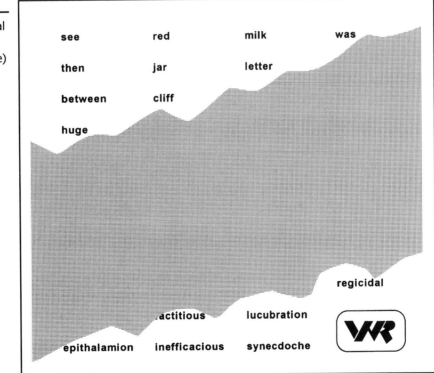

Alternate "stop" criteria for WRAT

Many patients, especially those with low literacy skills, may feel anxious when they see they are getting over their heads as the words on the WRAT 3 list become more difficult. They may recall the many times they felt badly in school when asked to read aloud. Yet the procedure requires them to continue the WRAT 3 test to the embarrassment of making 10 consecutive errors. The health care setting is a different environment than a classroom and they may feel demeaned and resentful. It may be worthwhile to trade off some of the precision attainable using the "10 stop" criterion (which was established for use in school systems) for the lesser precision required in most health care settings.

Adequate accuracy can be obtained when you stop the test after five errors in a row. Using the "stop at five" criterion, the error is less than one grade level compared to going all the way to 10 errors in a row.[9] The precision of the test can be further improved. After patients have made five errors in a row, ask them to look ahead to see if there are additional words they can pronounce. If any are found these are added to the patients' scores.

The REALM Test (Rapid Estimate of Adult Literacy in Medicine)

This test is similar to the WRAT test and correlates quite well with WRAT in terms of reading scores.[10,11] However, in the REALM, the patient reads from a list of 66 health/medical–related words. The REALM test words are arranged in three columns beginning with short easy words like *fat, flu,* and *pill,* proceeding to more difficult words like *medication* and *osteoporosis.* (See Figure 3-3 for word list.)

To administer the test, patients are asked to read the words in the three word lists aloud, starting at the top of List 1. The tester uses a corresponding word list to check the words pronounced correctly. When patients can read no further, they are asked to look down the lists and to pronounce any other words that they can. The raw score is the total number of words pronounced correctly. Table 3-1 can be used to convert the raw score into reading grade range.

REALM has several advantages over WRAT and other graded word tests. A principal advantage is that it is more likely to be accepted by patients in a health care setting because it uses medical and health-related words. Administration of REALM takes less time than WRAT. A third advantage is that the scoring is simpler. The fact that REALM offers less precision (scores are given as a *range* of grade levels rather than a specific grade level as in WRAT) is of little consequence for most health care purposes.

The REALM test, scoring guide, and a summary of validation results are given in Appendix B. Although REALM is a copyrighted test, there is no charge or cost to use or copy the test, provided that acknowledgment is given. A plastic enclosed REALM word list is available for a small fee from the REALM authors.

Should the reading skill of every patient be routinely tested by hospitals and clinics? Some hospitals already do this and enter patients' reading scores on their medical records. One reason in favor of testing every patient is to respond (partially) to the JCAHO patient education requirements. Another reason is to provide the hospital staff with information to help them select the materials and teaching methods most appropriate for each patient. Three reasons against testing the literacy skills of every patient are:

List 1	List 2	List 3
fat	fatigue	allergic
flu	pelvic	menstrual
pill	jaundice	testicle
dose	infection	colitis
eye	exercise	emergency
stress	behavior	medication
smear	prescription	occupation
nerves	notify	sexually
germs	gallbladder	alcoholism
meals	calories	irritation
disease	depression	constipation
cancer	miscarriage	gonorrhea
caffeine	pregnancy	inflammatory
attack	arthritis	diabetes
kidney	nutrition	hepatitis
hormones	menopause	antibiotics
herpes	appendix	diagnosis
seizure	abnormal	potassium
bowel	syphilis	anemia
asthma	hemorrhoids	obesity
rectal	nausea	osteoporosis
incest	directed	impetigo

SCORE

List 1 _____
List 2 _____
List 3 _____
Raw
Score _____

TABLE 3-1
REALM scoring chart

RAW SCORE	GRADE RANGE
0–18	3rd grade and below
19–44	4th to 6th grades
45–60	7th to 8th grades
61–66	9th grade and above

1. Unless the hospital staff is trained to apply appropriate teaching methods for each reading level, it cannot make effective use of the patients' literacy record.
2. Patients may initiate litigation if they believe that the hospital has made an unauthorized release of their literacy test results. Also, some low literacy patients may elect to seek medical services elsewhere upon learning of the literacy test and that it would be a permanent part of their medical record.
3. It adds to the overhead costs of the hospital.

Other reading tests

A number of other oral reading tests are in use in school systems. Among these are the Slosson Oral Reading Test (SORT) and the Peabody Individual Achievement Test–Revised (PIAT–R).[12,13] The SORT uses a series of word lists, each one scaled for a different grade level. The PIAT is an individually administered test to diagnose reading problems. Both of these tests may be used with patients, but the tests involve more procedural steps and they are likely to be more time consuming than the WRAT or REALM.

Neither the WRAT nor the REALM is available in other languages, but a Spanish version of WRAT is currently in the validation phase and may be available during 1995. Other languages employ different rules for pronunciation compared to English. Thus, a test in another language is not simply a matter of translating existing word lists into that language.

Using test results to select teaching methods

The results of word recognition tests of individuals or patient populations are useful criteria for selecting teaching methods. Box 3-2 presents a set of such teaching criteria. Additional criteria and teaching tips are found in Chapter 9.

The criteria in Box 3-2 offer only general guidelines for teaching methods, but are indicative of the benefits of applying these tests with your patient population.

Part 2: Reading Comprehension Testing Methods

Comprehension tests differ in design from reading tests (WRAT and REALM) in that the test instrument is based on a specific text passage that you may select rather than standard word lists. For that reason, comprehension tests

---

BOX 3-2

Teaching methods based on WRAT scores

> BELOW 5TH-GRADE SCORES
>
> — Use participative methods such as demonstration or discussion (see Chapter 9, Tips on Teaching).
> — Use short audiotapes, videotapes, single-concept flip charts.
> — Consider "end-use" teaching materials. For example, teach nutrition via shopping lists or restaurant menus rather than the food groups.
>
> BETWEEN 5TH AND 9TH GRADES
>
> — Use above methods plus pamphlets, booklets with low reading levels.
> — Use record-keeping diaries.
>
> 9TH GRADE AND ABOVE
>
> — Use all of the above plus simple charts and diagrams that include directions for use.

indicate the patient's reading skills *for the specific material used*. Thus, comprehension tests don't directly indicate patients' reading skills in terms of grade level—the test only indicates whether or not they can understand the specific pamphlet or booklet used in the test. This is an important distinction.

In comparison, reading tests such as WRAT and REALM do not require that patients understand the words—only that they are able to pronounce them. Subject matter is an important variable in reading comprehension. For example, an auto mechanic can read and understand material on carburetors with much greater ease than can a musician; in turn, a musician will find that the terms used in music make perfect sense whereas the auto mechanic may only shake his head.

For most people in the United States, health care subjects are not among their most familiar topics. Health instructions that appear to be straightforward to health care providers may not be understood by patients. A reading comprehension test is one way to measure how much is understood.

The Cloze Test

The Cloze test may be used for patients who have a WRAT/REALM score at the 6th grade or higher. Below the 6th grade the listening test should be used. Since the Cloze is a paper and pencil test, it is possible to administer it to a group of patients, but in practice it is usually administered to patients individually.

The Cloze test determines, directly, the fit between reader and material. The material may or may not be familiar to the reader. The test brings the reader and the material together with the task of filling in a series of blanks.Developed by Taylor (1953), the test is designed so that every fifth word is deleted from a passage, and the reader's task is to fill in the blanks with the exact replacements.[14] The ability of readers to fill in missing words correctly is a valid indicator of how well they understand the passage.

The Cloze test measures comprehension in two ways: (1) it tests how much knowledge was obtained from the information surrounding the blanks, and (2) it determines how well this information was used to obtain additional information.[15]

To use the Cloze, make up your own Cloze test from one or more of your frequently used health care materials. Detailed directions for making up a Cloze test are given in the following pages. Ideally, your Cloze test should have about 50 blanks for the patient to fill in.

For example, if you are a nurse working with patients who have chronic obstructive pulmonary disease (COPD), you might want to test your patients' ability to understand one of the instructions they are given. You might make up a Cloze test from one of your materials, such as the example shown in Figure 3-4. The example shows only a partial passage as it contains only 17 blanks, about one-third of the 50 blanks recommended.

The exact replacement words in Figure 3-4 are: *cough, those, prescription, your, make, you, sputum, this, from, easily, lung, even, bought, be, taking, prescribed, sure.*

FIGURE 3-4

Partial sample of a Cloze test

> ## CONTROL OF CHRONIC OBSTRUCTIVE PULMONARY DISEASE (COPD)
>
> ### Medications
>
> The pharmacist will explain the correct way to take the medication your doctor has prescribed for you.
>
> Do not take any _____ or cold remedies, including _____ you buy without a _____, without first checking with _____ doctor. These medications can _____ it more difficult for _____ to cough up the _____ from your lungs. If _____ sputum is not removed _____ your lungs, you can _____ get a respiratory or _____ infection.
>
> Remember, mixing medications _____ those that can be_____ without a prescription, can _____ dangerous. If you are _____ medications that have been _____ for other reasons, be _____ to inform your doctor.

Constructing and administering a Cloze test

To construct a Cloze test for your patients, select a manual, booklet, or other written instruction of some length (300 words or more) with contents of fairly even difficulty. Choose a passage that consists of prose that does not include lists, charts, or illustrations.

1. Leave the first sentence intact. Beginning with the second sentence, delete every fifth word until you have about 50 words deleted. Replace each word with a blank line; make all lines of equal length. Do not delete proper nouns (names); instead delete the word that follows the proper noun.

2. After introducing the test to the patient, explain the Cloze test by saying,

   > Here is an instruction that has some words left out. From the words that are there, see if you can fill in the missing word. If you get stuck, go on and come back later if you wish. Perhaps more than one word will make sense, but choose the word that seems best to you. Don't worry if you can't get them all. Hardly anyone does.

3. After the patient has filled in the words, compare the result with a copy of the original. Count as correct the words that are *exactly* like the original. Do not count any word other than the original, even if the substituted word makes sense. (The scoring allows for up to 40 percent of such substitutions without indicating a deficiency in reading skill.) Errors in word endings such as *s, ed,* and *ing* are counted as incorrect.

4. *Scoring the Cloze:* Determine the percentage correct by dividing the number of exact word replacements by the total number of blanks. For example:

39 correct replacements in 50 blanks
39 divided by 50 = .78 or 78% correct.

Interpreting the score:

Score (% exact replacements)	Interpretation
60–100%	The passage is understood. It should be easy for the patient.
40–59%	The material can be used but may require supplemental teaching.
below 40%	Not understood; not suitable.

Using Cloze results

We do not suggest that Cloze be administered to every patient in a hospital or clinic, but rather to a representative sample of patients. It might be administered to an individual patient who seems to be having difficulty understanding one of your health instruction materials. The authors have found that it takes about an hour or two to construct a Cloze test, and 10 to 20 minutes to test each patient. This is time well spent because the Cloze can verify that a patient understands— a key requirement of the new JCAHO directives mentioned early in this chapter.

If a significant number of your patients score below 40 percent on the Cloze test, the material used in the test is not appropriate for them. These patients need to be taught using a different method (see Chapter 9, Tips on Teaching), or the material used in the Cloze test must be revised. A clue as to what needs to be revised can be obtained by examining the completed Cloze tests to see which portions of the test caused the greatest number of errors.

A further clue as to how to revise the wording of the material to make it more understandable may be given in the *choice* of "wrong" words (not exact replacement words) that some patients wrote in the blanks. Those "wrong" words may be the more common expressions that are understood by your patient population, and if not incorrect in terms of the context of the material, they should be used in its revision. Additional characteristics of the material that may be the causes of difficulty may be uncovered by analyzing the material using the SAM instrument described in Chapter 4.

Listening tests for comprehension

The Cloze test is likely to prove too difficult for patients with reading skills below the 6th-grade level (approximately competency level 1 on NALS scale). Patients at this reading skill level lack fluency and read with hesitancy so the meanings of sentences and the context around the missing words (blanks) are likely to be elusive. A listening test may be required to test their comprehension skills. That is, you read a passage; the patient listens; you ask questions verbally and record the answers.

To construct the listening test, select the key points of the text—especially points dealing with desired behaviors—and write short questions on these (not more than 10). The selected text should not take longer than about 3 minutes to read. If it is longer than that, break it into segments with a reading and short question session for each segment.

The same scoring percentages used for Cloze have been used to score levels of comprehension from a listening test.[16] You may use any of your patient education materials that have readability levels below the 5th-grade level for a listening test. An illustrative listening test prepared from materials available to patients at the Norfolk, Virginia, Public Health Hospital is given in Box 3-3.

Administration of a short listening comprehension test takes less than 10 minutes. An additional advantage of the listening test is that besides its comprehension measurement, it opens the door for dialogue with patients and further questions they may have.

BOX 3-3

Sample passage for a listening comprehension test

Getting Flu Shots: Most people see a doctor when they are sick. When you are sick, it's easy to forget about the shots that could keep you from getting sick. Please listen to this, and if you need any shots or have any questions, see your doctor.

The Flu: For a lot of people the flu isn't a very bad illness, but some people get very sick with it and may even die from it. If you are one of these people who can get very sick from it, you should get a flu shot every year.

If you have not had a flu shot, talk to your doctor. You should have a flu shot if:
1. You are 65 years old or older.
2. You have diabetes, or lung, heart, kidney, or liver trouble, or if you've had another disease for a long time.

SAMPLE QUESTIONS FOR LISTENING TEST

Q-1. *According to what I've just read to you, why don't some people get their flu shots?*
A-1. Because they only see the doctor when they are already sick.

Q-2. *What should a person do if he thinks he needs a flu shot, or any other shot?*
A-2. See his doctor.

Q-3. *How long does a flu shot protect you?*
A-3. About a year (or, You need one every Fall).

Q-4. *What diseases make you more likely to need a flu shot?*
A-4. Diabetes, or lung, heart, kidney, liver, or any disease you've had a long time. (Any three count as a correct answer.)

Q-5. *At what age should older people have a flu shot?*
A-5. 65.

Summary

National literacy surveys provide extensive statistics on reading ability of the U.S. population as a whole, by ethnic group, and by age. Although these are useful data, they may or may not be representative of your patient population. Information on the reading level for your population can be quickly obtained by testing a sample of that population using word recognition tests such as WRAT or REALM.

Results of the reading tests can be used to help you select appropriate teaching methods for your patient population, and as threshold criteria for other surveys or tests such as the Cloze test. A few hospitals and some substance abuse programs test all incoming patients using a word recognition test and the test scores are entered on the patients' records.

Reading comprehension testing is a step beyond reading word recognition testing and may be done using the Cloze or a listening test. Results from these tests apply only to the individuals tested and the material used in the test. That is, the Cloze assesses the "literacy fit" of a specific material to a specific patient. Furthermore, the test can provide verification that your health care organization meets the patient comprehension requirements set forth by JCAHO for accreditation.

Applying this chapter in your practice: the next 90 days

Here are some ways you can apply the information learned in this chapter during the next 90 days that will make a difference in the way that you teach your patients. Even a very busy health professional has time to take one or two of the following actions.

With a colleague, take 20 minutes to practice administering the WRAT or REALM so you feel comfortable doing it. In your practice sessions, include giving the brief introduction and explanation of the test to the "patient."

- Administer the WRAT or REALM to 10 patients. Share the results with your colleagues.
- Based on the WRAT or REALM scores, decide on one new or different approach you will use to improve patient comprehension of your instructions.
- Construct a Cloze test from one of your most frequently used written health instructions. Use the Cloze to test three to ten patients. (First, use WRAT or REALM to screen for patients that are reading at least at the 6th-grade level.)
- From the test results, decide what changes are needed in the instruction you used for the Cloze test.

References

1. Doak C, Doak L (1980): Patient comprehension profiles: Recent findings and strategies. Patient Counselling and Health Education 2(3), third quarter.
2. Kirsh IS, Jungeblut A, Jenkins L, Kolstad A (1993): Adult Literacy in America. National Center for Education Statistics, U.S. Department of Education, p. xv.
3. Assessing Literacy: The Framework for the National Adult Literacy Survey (October 1992): Sup. of Documents, Mail Stop SSOP, Washington, DC 20402-9328, ISBN 0-16-038248-3.
4. Meade CD, Byrd JC (February 1989): Patient literacy and readability of smoking education literature. APHA Journal 79:204–206.
5. Wide Range Achievement Test (WRAT 3) (1993): Wide Range Inc., 1526 Gilpin Ave., Wilmington, DE 19806.
6. Hosey G, Freeman W, Stracqualursi F, Gohdes D (1990): Designing and evaluating diabetes education materials for American Indians. The Diabetes Educator 16:407–414.
7. Davis TC, Crouch MA, Wills G, et al. (1990): The gap between patient reading comprehension and the readability of patient education materials. Journal of Family Practice 31:533–538.
8. Jackson RF, Davis TC, Bairnsfather LE, Gault H (1991): Patient reading ability: an overlooked problem in health care. Southern Medical Journal 84(10):1172–1175.
9. Wilder L, Becker D (1993): Errors associated with WRAT test stopping criteria. Unpublished paper, Johns Hopkins Medical School.
10. Murphy, Peggy (source person for a copy of the REALM test). Department of Internal Medicine, Louisiana State University (MC-S), PO Box 33932, Shreveport, LA 71130-3932.
11. Murphy PW, Davis TC, et al. (October 1993): Rapid estimate of adult literacy in medicine (REALM): a quick reading test for patients. Journal of Reading 37(2):124–130.
12. Slosson RL (1990): Slosson oral reading test (SORT) revised. Slosson Educational Publications, 538 Buffalo Rd., East Aurora, NY 14052.
13. Markwardt FC. Peabody Individual Achievement Test. American Guidance Service, Circle Pine, MN.
14. Taylor, Wison (Fall, 1953): Cloze Procedure: A New Tool for Measuring Readability. Journalism Quarterly 30:415–433. The term *Cloze* was coined from the Gestalt concept of closure, a way to form a complete whole by filling in the gaps in the structure.
15. McKenna MC, Robinson RD (1980): An Introduction to the Cloze Procedure: An Annotated Bibliography, rev. ed. Newark, DE: International Reading Association.
16. McNeal B, et al. (May/June 1984): Comprehension assessment of diabetes education program participants. South Carolina diabetes control project. Department of Health and Environmental Control, Diabetes Care, p. 33, Columbia, SC.

4

"What is the best way to be sure that the materials are suitable for my patients?"

Assessing Suitability of Materials

How suitable are your patient education materials? Are your patients likely to understand them? To accept them? This chapter describes practical ways to analyze the suitability of materials so you can continue to use them with confidence, or have evidence of the need for revision. Another method for evaluation—using patients to assess suitability of materials—is given in Chapter 10, under Learner Verification and Revision of Materials.

An Overview of Testing Methods

The need to assess the suitability of materials has been with us for a long time. Text readability formulas made their appearance during the 1920s and received much elaboration over the next seven decades.[1] Flesch (1946) offered a mathematical "yardstick" for written materials based on the number of words, sentences, affixes, and personal references.[2] Jonassen (1982) suggests a 20-step evaluation process for books and booklets that relies on elaboration theory.[3] The U.S. Department of Agriculture, WIC nutrition program (1991), presents a 23-item evaluation list for text, and a 21-item list for audiovisual materials.[4] Wileman (1993) addresses visual design evaluation via a 13-point checklist.[5]

Recent reports from the National Adult Literacy Surveys (NALS) briefly explain the criteria to rate the difficulty of written materials used in the literacy testing of the US population.[6] Unfortunately, the NALS reports offer no easy-to-use "formula" suitable to rate health care pamphlets or booklets to score them on the 0 to 500 scale.

Computer-aided instruction (CAI), multimedia, hypertext, hypermedia: these instructional formats may be helpful in teaching patients with low literacy skills. How can patient education materials in these media be assessed? At this point the reader may be thinking, "Why bother? I don't even know what these all mean, and I don't use them to teach patients." We would respond that, perhaps not today, but with the forces of technology and cost containment advancing so rapidly, you can expect to be using at least some of these media within the next few years. These media are evolving so rapidly they present a difficult moving target for any one evaluation method. Although Skinner (1993) offers guidelines for selecting CAI programs, and Thompson (1992) presents a list of factors to consider in learning displays, a widely agreed upon assessment method is yet to be developed.[7,8]

For this chapter, the authors have selected the most practical current assessment methods. The following three easy-to-learn methods can be used to assess the difficulty and suitability of patient education materials:

1.   A checklist of attributes
2.   Analysis via readability formulas
3.   Analysis using SAM (Suitability Assessment of Materials), a new instrument

The three methods progress from an informal checklist of attributes of print materials to a more rigorous and quantified evaluation of materials in any medium using SAM. Before using any new patient instruction, health educators should consider assessing it using at least one of these methods.

An assessment using the checklist takes less than 15 minutes. Readability formulas can be learned and applied in 10 to 15 minutes and provide a grade-level measure of the reading difficulty of a material. The SAM instrument can be used immediately after reading the directions and takes 30 to 45 minutes to apply to a material. By acquiring the skills presented in this chapter you will be able to answer, with confidence, the following kinds of questions:

•   What is the reading difficulty of this written health material? Is the reading level too difficult for my patients?
•   Due to budget cuts, I can afford to order quantities of only one new pamphlet. I must select one that is suitable for nearly all my patients. Among the many offered, which one should I buy?
•   How can I assess materials for a wide range of suitability factors, including cultural factors?
•   How can I decide on the suitability of video- and audiotaped instructions?

An Assessment Checklist

The 17-item checklist (Figure 4-1) is one of the easiest and quickest ways to assess appropriateness of a material for patients. If you have to make a selection among a number of health care instructions, the list offers a quick way to screen to sort out the good from the not so good.

FIGURE 4-1

Checklist for print materials. (*Source:* Area Health Education Center, Biddeford, Maine)

Title of material:_____

Directions: Place a check next to each item that meets the described attribute.

ORGANIZATION

- ❏ 1. The cover is attractive. It indicates the core content and intended audience.
- ❏ 2. Desired behavior changes are stressed. "Need to know" information is stressed.
- ❏ 3. Not more than three or four main points are presented.
- ❏ 4. Headers and summaries are used to show organization and provide message repetition.
- ❏ 5. A summary that stresses what to do is included.

WRITING STYLE

- ❏ 6. The writing is in conversational style, active voice.
- ❏ 7. There is little or no technical jargon.
- ❏ 8. Text is vivid and interesting. Tone is friendly.

APPEARANCE:

- ❏ 9. Pages or sections appear uncluttered. Ample white spaces.
- ❏10. Lowercase letters used (capitals used only where grammatically needed).
- ❏11. There is a high degree of contrast between the print and the paper.
- ❏12. Print size is at least 12 point, serif type, and no stylized letters.
- ❏13. Illustrations are simple—preferably line drawings.
- ❏14. Illustrations serve to amplify the text.

APPEAL

- ❏15. The material is culturally, gender, and age appropriate.
- ❏16. The material closely matches the logic, language, and experience of the intended audience.
- ❏17. Interaction is invited via questions, responses, suggested action, etc.

As you read the material to be assessed, check off each of the attributes in Figure 4-1 found in the material. Any that are missing will indicate a potential deficiency in suitability. If the material is in the draft phase it can be revised. If the material has already been published and cannot easily be revised, the deficiencies point to where supplemental teaching may be required.

When using the checklist in Figure 4-1, you may find that some parts of the material possess an attribute, while other parts do not. For example, when considering item 13 on the checklist, one illustration might be simple and easy to understand, but another might be a copy from a medical textbook and far too complex. Resolve the dilemma on the basis of how important the illustrations are. If the complex illustration is *not* essential to understanding the key points of the material, then it does less harm and this favorable attribute on illustrations can be checked.

Readability Formulas

Readability formulas offer the health care provider an easy-to-use method to assess the reading difficulty of most print materials. In this section you will learn to use a readability formula.

What do they measure?

Readability formulas can be applied to prose—that is, running text—but not to tables, charts, or word lists. At least 40 different readability formulas are reported in the literature. Most of the 40 formulas are based on just two factors: word difficulty and sentence length. These formulas say that: "The greater the number of multi-syllable words, the greater the reading difficulty. Also, the longer the sentences, the greater the reading difficulty." Differences among the many formulas are mostly in the sample size and in the mathematical coefficients applied to the two factors.

Application of these two factors in a readability formula provides a grade-level rating. You can then compare the readability level of the material(s) with the reading skills of your patient population to determine suitability. (See Chapter 1 for data on literacy; Chapter 3 for methods to measure the reading skills of your patients.)

Knowing how to determine the readability level of your materials is critical to you and to your patients. You cannot afford to "fly blind." As noted in Chapter 1, the authors have found that health materials at college levels are often given to all patients—including those who have low and marginal reading skills. (See also Figure 6-1 in Chapter 6.) Is it any wonder that patients do not understand? That they do not follow directions for taking medications? That they miss their appointments?

Assessing readability using the Fry formula

Nearly all the 40+ readability formulas provide a reasonably accurate grade level (typically plus or minus one grade level with a 68-percent confidence factor). Among these formulas, the authors recommend the Fry formula. The Fry is widely accepted in the reading literature and among reading professionals and is not copyrighted. This formula applies from grade 1 through grade 17, and compared to some formulas, the Fry does not require as extensive a test sample.

It is not necessary to test the readability of every word and sentence. This would be especially tedious in a long booklet. Instead, test three samples from different parts of the instruction. For a very long text, such as a book of 50 pages or more, double the number to six samples.

Select a piece of material that you customarily use with your patients/clients and follow the five steps given below to determine its reading level using the Fry formula.[9]

Detailed directions

1. **Select three 100-word passages from the material you wish to test.** Count out exactly 100 words for each passage, starting with the first word of a sentence. (Omit headings.) If you are testing a very short pamphlet that may have only a few hundred words, select a single 100-word sample to test.

    Readability levels may vary considerably from one part of your material to another. Therefore, select the three samples from different content topics, if possible. For example, if a pamphlet includes such topics as the disease process, treatment options, and actions the patient should take, select one sample from each of these topics.

    Additional information:

    - Count proper nouns. Hyphenated words count as one word.
    - A word is defined as a group of symbols with a space on either side; thus "IRA," "1994," and "&" are each one word.

2. **Count the number of *sentences* in each 100 words, estimating the fractional length of the last sentence to the nearest 1/10.** For example, if the 100th word occurs 5 words into a 15-word sentence, the fraction of the sentence is 5/15 or 1/3 or 0.3.

3. **Count the total number of *syllables* in each 100-word passage.** You can count by making a small check mark over each syllable. For initializations (e.g., IRA) and numerals (e.g., 1994), count 1 syllable for each symbol. So "IRA" = 3 syllables and "1994" = 4 syllables.

    There is a short cut to counting the syllables. Since each 100-word sample must have at least 100 syllables, skip the first syllable in each word. Don't count it; just add 100 after you finish the count. Count only the remaining syllables (that are greater than one) in the 100-word sample. Thus, you don't put check marks over any of the one-syllable words; you put only one check over each two-syllable word, two checks over three-syllable words, and so forth.

    Occasionally you may be in doubt as to the number of syllables in a word. Resolve the doubt by placing a finger under your chin, say the word aloud, and count the number of times your chin drops. Each chin drop counts as a syllable.

4. **Calculate the average number of sentences and the average number of syllables from the three passages.** This is done by dividing the totals obtained from the three samples by 3 as shown in the example below.

Example:

	NUMBER OF SENTENCES	NUMBER OF SYLLABLES
1st 100 words	5.9	124
2nd 100 words	4.8	141
3rd 100 words	6.1	158
Totals	*16.8*	*423*
Divide Totals by 3:	5.6 Average	141 Average

5. **Refer to the Fry graph.** On the horizontal axis, find the line for the *average number of syllables* (141 for above example). On the vertical axis find the line for the *average number of sentences* (5.6 for the example). The readability grade level of the material is found at the point where the two lines intersect.

In the example above, the Fry chart shows the readability level at the 8th grade (see dot at the intersection in Figure 4-2). The curved line through the center of the Fry graph shows the locus of greatest accuracy. With a little practice, the five-step process will become much easier. You will soon be able to determine a readability level in less than 10 minutes.

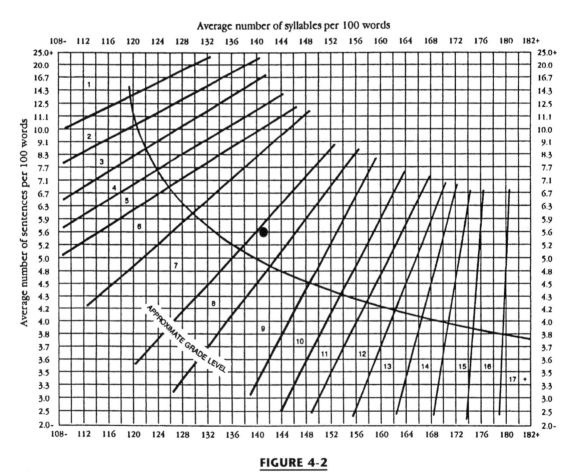

FIGURE 4-2

Fry graph for estimating readability—extended

Readability formulas: an important predictor

Fry and other readability authorities point out that the formulas predict the level of reading difficulty, but not all of the causes. The two factors assessed by the formulas, long sentences and difficult vocabulary, are recognized as only two among many. Nonetheless, the formulas are widely used and are an important predictor of overall suitability of patient instructions.

The authors have found a strong correlation between the readability level and the SAM instrument described later in this chapter. Although readability level is only one of the 22 SAM factors, it is pivotal. If readability is high (difficult), the overall SAM score is usually low (less suitable). The converse is also true.

Readability assessment by computer programs

At this writing, at least a dozen computer programs are on the market to assess readability.[10,11] The cost of these programs is less than US$100 each. If you have one of these computer programs, you can obtain a readability measure at the stroke of a key for any text material stored in the computer. The programs provide a range of other useful information as well. They may indicate violations of grammar rules such as a noun-verb mismatch, style rules such as active/passive voice, usage rules such as legalese, lists of "uncommon" words, and punctuation rules such as unnecessary or missing commas. They may suggest alternative words for you to consider and most of them offer corrected spelling.

For materials not already stored in your computer, it may be quicker to use the Fry formula as described above rather than to type the text into your computer.

Readability formulas for other languages

Readability formulas for text are currently available in at least 12 languages other than English. The languages include Chinese, Danish, Dutch, French, German, Hebrew, Hindi, Korean, Russian, Spanish, Swedish, and Vietnamese. For many of these languages, especially Spanish and German, you have a choice among several formulas.

The two variables used in formulas for English-language text, the number of syllables and length of the sentences, are used in most formulas for other languages as well. Some of these employ additional variables such as the number of words that separate the subject from the verb. Zakaluk and Samuels (1988) provide guidance on the selection and use of these formulas.[12]

A readability goal for your instructions

You may ask, "What is a reasonable readability goal? How low does it have to be?" The answer is to make it as low as practical without sacrificing important content or writing style. It is better to use conversational writing style even though you might squeeze your text a little lower on the readability scale using short, choppy sentences. Write for the patient, not for the formula.

The 6th-grade level is a reasonable goal for most health care instructions. About 75 percent of adult Americans will be able to read at this level without difficulty. If you want to make the instruction easily readable by 90 percent of adult Americans, it must be written at about the 3rd-grade level. Methods and examples of writing at low readability levels are presented in Chapter 6.

A frequently asked question is, "But won't good readers feel talked down to by instructions that have a low reading level?" Frederickson (1994) and others have shown that adults at all reading skill levels prefer and learn better with easy-to-read instructions.[13]

Factors beyond the readability formulas

At this point it is well to mention some attributes of print materials that are not included in the formulas but affect reading difficulty. (These are included in the checklist presented in Figure 4-1 and in the SAM instrument shown in the following pages.) The attributes include:

- **The print size and type style.** Print size on some health care materials may be so small that it is readable only by those with good eyesight. (See Chapter 6, Writing the Message, for type styles that are easiest to read.)
- **Color contrast between the ink and the paper.** Some materials have hues of artistic appeal (brown ink on tan paper), but these provide poor contrast which makes reading difficult.
- **The self-efficacy factor.** Does it look hard to read? A page of solid text may, by its appearance alone, discourage any reader.
- **The concept density.** Are many concepts and facts jammed into each paragraph—even in paragraphs with low readability scores?
- **Unfamiliar context.** Medical and scientific contexts are not familiar milieus for millions of patients. The meaning of common words may not be understood when used in an unfamiliar context. This is illustrated in the example that follows—from outside the health care field.

Consider these common words:

squares	combined	within
variance	divided	estimate
degrees	interaction	cells
freedom	sums	circumstances

Taken separately, a good reader will probably know the meaning for each of these words. However, if these words appear in a text about statistics (like the one below), many good readers suddenly feel illiterate—at least on this subject.

Under certain circumstances the within-cells and the interaction sums of squares may be added together and divided by the combined degrees of freedom to obtain an estimate of the variance based on a larger number of degrees of freedom.

The sentence presents these words in an unfamiliar context for most of us, and includes a large number of concepts and facts as well. A parallel can be drawn from this statistical example to health instructions. In health messages, it is not only the medical or technical words that may cause trouble, but also the more common words when used in unfamiliar contexts.

Suitability Assessment of Materials (SAM)

A dilemma facing many health care providers is how to systematically assess the suitability of a health care instruction for a given patient population, and do it in the short time available. The authors recognize that an ideal way is to evaluate the instruction with a sample of the intended audience, but often there is neither time nor resources for that. The assessment must be made analytically "at your desk."

Our response to this dilemma was to develop and validate SAM: a suitability assessment of materials instrument.[14] Validation was conducted with 172 health care providers from several cultures.[15] The cultures included Southeast Asians, Native Americans, and African Americans as well as students and faculty from the University of North Carolina School of Public Health and Johns Hopkins School of Medicine.

SAM was originally designed for use with print material and illustrations, but it has also been applied successfully to video- and audiotaped instructions. For each material, SAM provides a numerical score (in percent) that may fall in one of three categories: superior, adequate, or not suitable.

There is a continuing need for more comprehensive evaluation instruments. For instance, one can expect that in the near future a computer program will be developed that will evaluate instructions in text, visuals, audio/verbal, interactive television, multimedia, and combinations of these. Until such a program is developed, SAM is a logical step toward meeting that need.

The application of SAM can pinpoint specific deficiencies in an instruction that reduce its suitability. If the material is still in its developmental stage, these deficiencies can be corrected. If the material is already in use, the deficiencies indicate what supplemental instructions (perhaps verbal explanations) are needed.

Using SAM to evaluate a health care instruction

To use SAM for the first time, follow the six steps below:

1. Read through the SAM factor list and the evaluation criteria.
2. Read the material (or view the video) you wish to evaluate and write brief statements as to its purpose(s) and key points.
3. For short instructions, evaluate the entire piece. For long instructions, select samples to evaluate.
4. Evaluate and score each of the 22 SAM factors.
5. Calculate total suitability score.
6. Decide on the impact of deficiencies and what action to take.

The entire process to evaluate your instructional material should take 30 to 45 minutes the first time through. For subsequent applications of SAM, you may skip the first step because the SAM factors and criteria will be already familiar to you.

For a first-time use of SAM, we suggest you test a simple, short material that has only a few illustrations.

1. **Read the SAM instrument and the evaluation criteria.**

2. **Read the material to be assessed.** Read (or view) the material you plan to evaluate. It will help if you write brief statements as to its purpose(s) and its key points. Refer to these as you evaluate each SAM factor. Use a note pad to jot down comments and observations as you read the material, view the video, or listen to the audiotape.

3. **The sampling process for SAM is somewhat similar to that described earlier for selecting samples to apply a readability formula.** If you are applying SAM to a short material such as a single-page instruction or a typical pamphlet (twofold or threefold), assess the entire instruction. Similarly, for audio- and videotaped instructions of less than 10 minutes, evaluate the entire instruction.

   To apply SAM to a longer text, such as a booklet, select three pages that deal with topics central to the purpose of the booklet. For booklets of more than 50 pages, increase the sample size to six pages. For video- or audiotaped instructions exceeding 10 minutes, select topics in 2-minute blocks from the beginning, middle, and end sections of the video or audio presentation.

4. **Evaluate material vs. criteria for each factor, decide on its rating, and record it on the score sheet.** As you seek to evaluate your material against each factor, you are likely to find wide variation among different parts of your material. For any one factor, some parts may rate high (superior) while other parts of the same material rate low (unsuitable). For example, some illustrations may include captions while others do not. Resolve this dilemma by giving most weight to the part of your material that includes the key points that you previously identified in step 2 above.

   Materials that meet the superior criteria for a factor are scored 2 points for that factor; adequate receives 1 point; not suitable receives a zero. For factors that do not apply, write N/A. Use the SAM scoring sheet shown in Figure 4-3 to record your score for each of the 22 factors and to guide you in calculating the overall rating in percent.

5. **Calculate the total suitability score.** When you have evaluated all the factors, and written a score for each one on the score sheet, add up the scores to obtain a total score. Spaces to do this are provided on the score sheet. The maximum possible total score is 44 points (100 percent)—a perfect rating, which almost never happens. A more typical example: if the total score for your material is 34, your percent score is 34/44 or 77 percent.

   For some instructional materials, one or more of the 22 SAM factors may not apply. For example, for an audiotape or a videotape, the text readability

FIGURE 4-3

SAM scoring sheet

2 points for superior rating
1 point for adequate rating
0 points for not suitable rating
N/A if the factor does not apply to this material

FACTOR TO BE RATED	SCORE	COMMENTS

1. CONTENT

(a) Purpose is evident   2   _____
(b) Content about behaviors   2   _____
(c) Scope is limited   1   _____
(d) Summary or review included   1   _____

2. LITERACY DEMAND

(a) Reading grade level   2   _____
(b) Writing style, active voice   2   _____
(c) Vocabulary uses common words   2   _____
(d) Context is given first   1   _____
(e) Learning aids via "road signs"   1   _____

3. GRAPHICS

(a) Cover graphic shows purpose   1   _____
(b) Type of graphics   1   _____
(c) Relevance of illustrations   1   _____
(d) List, tables, etc. explained   0   _____
(e) Captions used for graphics   0   _____

4. LAYOUT AND TYPOGRAPHY

(a) Layout factors   1   _____
(b) Typography   1   _____
(c) Subheads ("chunking") used   2   _____

5. LEARNING STIMULATION, MOTIVATION

(a) Interaction used   2   _____
(b) Behaviors are modeled and   2   _____
     specific
(c) Motivation—self-efficacy   2   _____

6. CULTURAL APPROPRIATENESS

(a) Match in logic, language,   2   _____
     experience
(b) Cultural image and examples   1   _____

Total SAM score:_____

Total possible score:_____, Percent score:_____%

level (factor 2a) does not apply. To account for SAM factors that occasionally may not apply to a particular material, subtract 2 points for each N/A from the 44 total. Let's do that using the example from the paragraph above. If you arrived at a total score of 34 as noted above, but had one N/A factor, subtract 2 points from 44 to a revised maximum score of 42. Thus, the percent rating would become 34/42, for a rating of 81 percent.

Interpretation of SAM percentage ratings:

70–100 percent	superior material
40–69 percent	adequate material
0–39 percent	not suitable material

6. **Evaluate the impact of deficiencies; decide on revisions.** A deficiency, especially an "unsuitable" rating, in any of the 22 factors is significant. Many of these can be readily overcome by revising a draft material or by adding a supplemental instruction to a material already published. However, factors in two of the groups, the readability level and cultural appropriateness, must be considered as potential go–no/go signals for suitability regardless of the overall rating.

For example, except in the rare cases where an instruction contains a set of illustrations that replicate the entire message given in the text, a written instruction with a very high readability level will not be understood and is unsuitable. Similarly, a material that portrays an ethnic group in an inappropriate way is almost surely unsuitable because it is likely to be rejected by members of that ethnic group.

SAM evaluation criteria

1. Content

A. PURPOSE

Explanation: It is important that readers/clients readily understand the intended purpose of the instruction for them. If they don't clearly perceive the purpose, they may not pay attention or may miss the main point.

Superior	Purpose is explicitly stated in title, or cover illustration, or introduction.
Adequate	Purpose is not explicit. It is implied, or multiple purposes are stated.
Not suitable	No purpose is stated in the title, cover illustration, or introduction.

B. CONTENT TOPICS

Explanation: Since adult patients usually want to solve their immediate health problem rather than learn a series of medical facts (that may only *imply* a solution), the content of greatest interest and use to clients is likely to be behavior information to help solve their problem.

Superior	Thrust of the material is application of knowledge/skills aimed at desirable reader behavior rather than nonbehavior facts.
Adequate	At least 40 percent of content topics focus on desirable behaviors or actions.
Not suitable	Nearly all topics are focused on nonbehavior facts.

C. SCOPE

Explanation: Scope is limited to purpose or objective(s). Scope is also limited to what the patient can reasonably learn in the time allowed.

Superior	Scope is limited to essential information directly related to the purpose. Experience shows it can be learned in time allowed.
Adequate	Scope is expanded beyond the purpose; no more than 40 percent is nonessential information. Key points can be learned in time allowed.
Not suitable	Scope is far out of proportion to the purpose and time allowed.

D. SUMMARY AND REVIEW

Explanation: A review offers the readers/viewers a chance to see or hear the key points of the instruction in other words, examples, or visuals. Reviews are important; readers often miss the key points upon first exposure.

Superior	A summary is included and retells the key messages in different words and examples.
Adequate	Some key ideas are reviewed.
Not suitable	No summary or review is included.

2. Literacy demand

A. READING GRADE LEVEL (FRY FORMULA)

Explanation: Unless the instruction presents the topics completely without text (via visual, demonstrations, and/or audio), the text reading level may be a critical factor in patient comprehension. Reading formulas can provide a reasonably accurate measure of reading difficulty.

Superior	5th-grade level or lower (5 years of schooling level).
Adequate	6th-, 7th-, or 8th-grade level (6–8 years of schooling level).
Not suitable	9th-grade level and above (9 years or more of schooling level).

B. WRITING STYLE

Explanation: Conversational style and active voice lead to easy-to-understand text. Example: "Take your medicine every day." Passive voice is less effective. Example: "Patients should be advised to take their medicine every day." Embedded information, the long or multiple phrases included in a sentence, slows down the reading process and generally makes comprehension more difficult.

Superior	Both factors: (1) Mostly conversational style and active voice. (2) Simple sentences are used extensively; few sentences contain embedded information.
Adequate	(1) About 50 percent of the text uses conversational style and active voice. (2)Less than half the sentences have embedded information.
Not suitable	(1) Passive voice throughout. (2)Over half the sentences have extensive embedded information.

c. Vocabulary

Explanation: Common, explicit words are used (for example, doctor vs. physician). The instruction uses few or no words that express general terms such as categories (for example, legumes vs. beans), concepts (for example, normal range vs. 15 to 70), and value judgments (for example, excessive pain vs. pain lasts more than 5 minutes). Imagery words are used because these are words people can "see" (for example, whole wheat bread vs. dietary fiber; a runny nose vs. excess mucus).

Superior	All three factors: (1) Common words are used nearly all of the time. (2) Technical, concept, category, value judgment (CCVJ) words are explained by examples. (3) Imagery words are used as appropriate for content.
Adequate	(1) Common words are frequently used. (2) Technical and CCVJ words are sometimes explained by examples. (3) Some jargon or math symbols are included.
Not suitable	Two or more factors: (1) Uncommon words are frequently used in lieu of common words. (2) No examples are given for technical and CCVJ words. (3) Extensive jargon.

d. In sentence construction, the context is given before new information

Explanation: We learn new facts/behaviors more quickly when told the context first. Good example: "To find out what's wrong with you (the context first), the doctor will take a sample of your blood for lab tests" (new information).

Superior	Consistently provides context before presenting new information.
Adequate	Provides context before new information about 50 percent of the time.
Not suitable	Context is provided last or no context is provided.

e. Learning enhancement by advance organizers (road signs)

Explanation: Headers or topic captions should be used to tell very briefly what's coming up next. These "road signs" make the text look less formidable, and also prepare the reader's thought process to expect the announced topic.

Superior	Nearly all topics are preceded by an advance organizer (a statement that tells what is coming next).
Adequate	About 50 percent of the topics are preceded by advance organizers.
Not suitable	Few or no advance organizers are used.

3. Graphics (illustrations, lists, tables, charts, graphs)

A. COVER GRAPHIC

Explanation: People *do* judge a booklet by its cover. The cover image often is the deciding factor in a patient's attitude toward, and interest in, the instruction.

Superior	The cover graphic is (1) friendly, (2) attracts attention, (3) clearly portrays the purpose of the material to the intended audience.
Adequate	The cover graphic has one or two of the superior criteria.
Not suitable	The cover graphic has none of the superior criteria.

B. TYPE OF ILLUSTRATIONS

Explanation: Simple line drawings can promote realism without including distracting details. (Photographs often include unwanted details.) Visuals are accepted and remembered better when they portray what is familiar and easily recognized. Viewers may not recognize the meaning of medical textbook drawings or abstract art/symbols.

Superior	Both factors: (1) Simple, adult-appropriate, line drawings/sketches are used. (2) Illustrations are likely to be familiar to the viewers.
Adequate	One of the superior factors is missing.
Not suitable	None of the superior factors are present.

C. RELEVANCE OF ILLUSTRATIONS

Explanation: Nonessential details such as room background, elaborate borders, unneeded color can distract the viewer. The viewer's eyes may be "captured" by these details. The illustrations should tell the key points visually.

Superior	Illustrations present key messages visually so the reader/viewer can grasp the key ideas from the illustrations alone. No distractions.
Adequate	(1) Illustrations include some distractions. (2) Insufficient use of illustrations.
Not suitable	One factor: (1) Confusing or technical illustrations (nonbehavior related). (2) No illustrations, or an overload of illustrations.

D. GRAPHICS: LISTS, TABLES, GRAPHS, CHARTS, GEOMETRIC FORMS

Explanation: Many readers do not understand the author's purpose for the lists, charts, and graphs. Explanations and directions are essential.

Superior	Step-by-step directions, with an example, are provided that will build comprehension and self-efficacy.
Adequate	"How-to" directions are too brief for reader to understand and use the graphic without additional counseling.
Not suitable	Graphics are presented without explanation.

E. CAPTIONS ARE USED TO "ANNOUNCE"/EXPLAIN GRAPHICS

Explanation: Captions can quickly tell the reader what the graphic is all about, where to focus within the graphic. A graphic without a caption is usually an inferior instruction and represents a missed learning opportunity.

Superior	Explanatory captions with all or nearly all illustrations and graphics.
Adequate	Brief captions used for some illustrations and graphics.
Not suitable	Captions are not used.

4. Layout and typography

A. LAYOUT

Explanation: Layout has a substantial influence on the suitability of materials.

Superior	At least five of the following eight factors are present:

1. Illustrations are on the same page adjacent to the related text.
2. Layout and sequence of information are consistent, making it easy for the patient to predict the flow of information.
3. Visual cuing devices (shading, boxes, arrows) are used to direct attention to specific points or key content.
4. Adequate white space is used to reduce appearance of clutter.
5. Use of color supports and is not distracting to the message. Viewers need not learn color codes to understand and use the message.
6. Line length is 30–50 characters and spaces.
7. There is high contrast between type and paper.
8. Paper has nongloss or low-gloss surface.

Adequate	At least three of the superior factors are present.
Not suitable	(1) Two (or less) of the superior factors are present. (2) Looks uninviting or discouragingly hard to read.

B. TYPOGRAPHY

Explanation: Type size and fonts can make text easy or difficult for readers at all skill levels. For example, type in ALL CAPS slows everybody's reading comprehension. Also, when too many (six or more) type fonts and sizes are used on a page, the appearance becomes confusing and the focus uncertain.

Superior   The following four factors are present:

1. Text type is in uppercase and lowercase serif (best) or sans-serif.
2. Type size is at least 12 point.
3. Typographic cues (bold, size, color) emphasize key points.
4. No ALL CAPS for long headers or running text.

Adequate   Two of the superior factors are present.

Not suitable   One or none of the superior factors are present. Or, six or more type styles and sizes are used on a page.

C. SUBHEADINGS OR "CHUNKING"

Explanation: Few people can remembering more than seven independent items. For adults with low literacy skills the limit may be three- to five-item lists. Longer lists need to be partitioned into smaller "chunks."

Superior   (1) Lists are grouped under descriptive subheadings or "chunks."
                  (2) No more than five items are presented without a subheading.

Adequate   No more than seven items are presented without a subheading.

Not suitable   More than seven items are presented without a subheading.

5. Learning stimulation and motivation

A. INTERACTION INCLUDED IN TEXT AND/OR GRAPHIC

Explanation: When the patient responds to the instruction—that is, does something to reply to a problem or question—chemical changes take place in the brain that enhance retention in long-term memory. Readers/viewers should be asked to solve problems, to make choices, to demonstrate, etc.

Superior   Problems or questions presented for reader responses.

Adequate   Question-and-answer format used to discuss problems and solutions (passive interaction).

Not suitable   No interactive learning stimulation provided.

B. DESIRED BEHAVIOR PATTERNS ARE MODELED, SHOWN IN SPECIFIC TERMS

Explanation: People often learn more readily by observation and by doing it themselves rather than by reading or being told. They also learn more readily when specific, familiar instances are used rather than the abstract or general.

Superior   Instruction models specific behaviors or skills. (For example, for nutrition instruction, emphasis is given to changes in eating patterns or shopping or food preparation/cooking tips; tips to read labels.)

Adequate	Information is a mix of technical and common language that the reader may not easily interpret in terms of daily living (for example: *Technical:* Starches—80 calories per serving; High Fiber—1–4 grams of fiber in a serving).
Not suitable	Information is presented in nonspecific or category terms such as the food groups.

c. Motivation

Explanation: People are more motivated to learn when they believe the tasks/behaviors are doable by them.

Superior	Complex topics are subdivided into small parts so that readers may experience small successes in understanding or problem solving, leading to self-efficacy.
Adequate	Some topics are subdivided to improve the readers' self-efficacy.
Not suitable	No partitioning is provided to create opportunities for small successes.

6. Cultural appropriateness

a. Cultural match: logic, language, experience (LLE)

Explanation: A valid measure of cultural appropriateness of an instruction is how well its logic, language, and experience (inherent in the instruction) match the LLE of the intended audience. For example, a nutrition instruction is a poor cultural match if it tells readers to eat asparagus and romaine lettuce if these vegetables are rarely eaten by people in that culture and are not sold in the readers' neighborhood markets.

Superior	Central concepts/ideas of the material appear to be culturally similar to the LLE of the target culture.
Adequate	Significant match in LLE for 50 percent of the central concepts.
Not suitable	Clearly a cultural mismatch in LLE.

b. Cultural image and examples

Explanation: To be accepted, an instruction must present cultural images and examples in realistic and positive ways.

Superior	Images and examples present the culture in positive ways.
Adequate	Neutral presentation of cultural images or foods.
Not suitable	Negative image such as exaggerated or caricatured cultural characteristics, actions, or examples.

In summary, the SAM offers a systematic method to assess suitability of materials. In about 30 minutes you can obtain a numerical suitability score that you can use to decide whether or not a material is suitable for your patient population.

When making an evaluation using SAM, or using the checklist presented earlier in this chapter, you may have uncovered one or more specific deficiencies. If so, decide on how critical the deficiencies are to patient comprehension and acceptance of the key messages of your material. Guidance for making this decision may be found in Chapters 2 and 5. To overcome the deficiencies, you will find specific details related to each instructional media in the following chapters: Chapter 6 for written materials, Chapter 7 for visuals and graphics, and Chapter 8 for videotapes, audiotapes, and multimedia.

Summary

The health care "culture" relies heavily on written instructions. These may be assessed by using a checklist of attributes that define easy-to-read materials. Another assessment worth making is to test the material using a readability formula. If you assess the readability and suitability of your health care instructions, you are more likely to provide instructions your patients will understand.

Materials that have readability levels of 9th grade or higher need to be rewritten to make them understandable by most Americans. If the materials are not rewritten, supplemental instruction will be needed by most patients when the material is used.

The suitability of a written material depends on many factors. Although readability formulas measure only a few of these characteristics, the reading level is usually a "go–no/go" criterion to predict patient comprehension of the material.

Consider using the SAM instrument to obtain a numerical rating that covers the many other suitability factors not included in readability formulas. SAM addresses suitability in terms of content, literacy demand, graphics, layout, learning stimulation/motivation, and culture of the intended audience.

It is important to note that the assessment methods presented in this chapter use analytical methods exclusively. Another method of assessment—using patients to test the suitability of the material—is presented in Chapter 10, Learner Verification and Revision (LVR) of Materials.

Actions you can take during the next 90 days

- Use the checklist to screen three of your frequently used health care instructions.
- Test the readability of 10 of your written health care materials and record the grade level on the back of each piece. Share this with your colleagues.
- Compare the readability levels of the 10 materials with the reading levels of the adult population of the United States by referring to literacy data in Figure 1-1. Determine how many of the 10 instructions are "over the heads" of at least half the U.S. adult population in terms of reading skills.
- Use the SAM instrument to evaluate the suitability of one of your frequently used health care instructions.

- Use the information from the actions above to fashion a response to the new JCAHO requirement directives for patient understanding.
- Form a small committee at your health care organization to evaluate all new health care instructions.

References

1. Zakaluk BL, Samuels SJ (1988): Readability: Its Past, Present & Future. Newark: DE: International Reading Association, pp 2–15.
2. Flesch R (1946): The Art of Plain Talk. New York: Harper & Row, pp. 58–65.
3. Jonassen DH (1982): The Technology of Text. Englewood Cliffs, NJ: Educational Technology Publications, pp 83–87.
4. Nutrition Education Resource Guide (1991): Pub. No. 94. National Agricultural Library, Beltsville, MD, Appendix A.
5. Wileman RE (1993): Visual Communicating. Englewood Cliffs, NJ: Educational Technology Publications, pp 120–121.
6. Kirsch I, et al. (1993): Adult Literacy in America. A first look at the results of the national adult literacy survey. U.S. Department of Education, pp. 8–9.
7. Skinner CS, et al. (1993): The Potential of Computers in Patient Education. Indiana University Medical Center, p. 10.
8. Thompson AD, Simonson MR, Hargrave CP (1992): Educational Technology: A Review of the Research. Washington, DC: Association for Educational Communication and Technology Press, p. 50.
9. Fry E (December 1977): Fry's readability graph: clarifications, validity, and extensions to level 17. Journal of Reading, pp. 242–252.
10. Readability Analysis (1992): Gamco Industries Inc., PO Box 1862N, Big Springs, TX 79721-9990. Provides results of three readability analyses: Spache, Dale-Chall, and Fry.
11. Readability Analysis: Teacher Resource. GAMCO Industries Inc., PO Box 1911H8, Big Springs, TX 79721-1911. Uses three formulas.
12. Zakaluk BL, Samuels SJ (1988): Readability: Its Past, Present, and Future. Newark, DE: International Reading Association, pp.46–76.
13. Frederickson D (May 4, 1994): Polio vaccine informational pamphlets: study of parent comprehension comparing a short polio vaccine information pamphlet containing graphics and simple language with the currently available Public Health Service brochure. Presented at the Ambulatory Pediatrics Association annual conference, Seattle, WA.
14. SAM was developed by the authors under the Johns Hopkins School of Medicine project "Nutrition Education in Urban African Americans" funded by the National Institutes of Health, National Heart, Lung and Blood Institute, Bethesda, MD, 1993.
15. Doak C, Doak L, Miller K, Wilder L (November 1, 1994): Suitability Assessment of Materials (SAM). American Public Health Association Annual Meeting, Washington, DC.

*"Our biggest problem...
does the patient <u>really</u>
understand?"*

The Comprehension Process

It is not surprising that, "Do you understand?" is one of the most common questions in patient-care settings. It is essential that patients understand how to carry out their regimen. This chapter describes the conditions necessary for remembering and learning.

Comprehension is a complex process that depends on the effective interaction of logic, language, and experience as well as other factors. Comprehension results in grasping the meaning of the instruction.

To make this chapter more meaningful, we suggest you select a sample of one of your own teaching materials—perhaps a pamphlet or page that patients seem to have difficulty learning. Keep this at hand as you read this chapter, and as you progress we'll ask you to consider how this material could be made easier to learn.

The Memory System

Simply described, our memory may be seen as having three main processing systems: sensory information processing, short-term memory, and long-term memory. As with computers, our mental systems deal with information collection, storage, and retrieval. And like computers, each memory component has a capacity limit, a storage time limit, and specific procedures if storage and retrieval are to take place. It is most helpful to know these limits if our teaching is to result in patient learning.

Getting your message into the patient's memory systems

Gaining Attention: The starting point in comprehension is gaining the patient's attention. Why is this so important? Gaining attention "turns on" the electrical connections and initiates the necessary chemical changes that transport messages within the brain. You can do this by vividly telling patients the benefits they can receive by listening to what you have to say, by reading the pamphlet, or listening to a tape, or viewing a video. This helps gain their attention. The patient has to activate his own memory system by paying attention.

The initial processing: How can you help at this stage? Since the communications signal comes from the five senses, involve as many of these senses as possible so that the message is reinforced. Show a picture, read a piece of text, demonstrate so that if the message doesn't come through one way, it will have a second chance by another route.

The real difficulty at this stage of the memory system is that further information processing is not automatic. It only occurs when the mind pays attention to the signal and gives it a priority. Do I like it? Do I want it? Do I need to pay attention to this?

Assuming you've captured the patient's attention, how do you get your message into her short-term memory?

Getting through the short-term memory

Short-term memory has two characteristics that affect all of us:

1. It has a very *limited capacity.*
2. It has a *short storage time.*

In well-educated and well-trained adults, short-term memory can rarely store more than seven independent items at one time.[1] Our minds have much in common with a computer shift register that has just seven slots for short-term data storage. If more than seven independent items vie for our memory—such as steps in a medical procedure, or items on a diet list—the arrival of the eighth piece of information causes the human shift register to say, "Dump!" Then all seven slots may be wiped out in preparation to receive the next items of information.

The message for us all is that if we present lists with more than seven items, people not only don't remember the items beyond number seven, but they lose all or most of the first seven as well! Perhaps you've heard a colleague say,

"Well, they may not learn all these (15 items), but I'll include them all. They should get some of it."

Not true! *The more you include, the less they remember.* For people who have had less education and training, they may remember less than seven items; perhaps five or fewer may be their current working limit. At this point we ask you to review the material you selected at the start of this chapter. Does it present more than seven independent items for patients? If it does, it won't get through their short-term memories, and will not be remembered.

Perhaps you've experienced this limitation at a meeting or party when you were introduced to many new people. You meet one person after another; you smile and exchange names. When you have met them all you are dismayed that you remember few if any of the names! The information is forgotten because of a memory overload. If you doubt this memory limitation, read the easy words listed below, then close the book and attempt to write them down. Then reopen the book and see how many you could recall correctly.

this	getting	can
five	of	vegetables
risk	fruits	your
and	cancer	eat
day	a	cut

A more appropriate way to teach these 15 words without overtaxing our limited memory is by "chunking" the 15 items so they will fit within the limits of short-term memory. Chunking is a process of regrouping like information into several, smaller groups. Each of the smaller groups is "chunked" under its own descriptive subheader. For example, the 15 words could be chunked into two short sentences—just two "items" for our seven-item short-term memory capacity to cope with. "Eat five fruits and vegetables a day. This can cut your risk of getting cancer."

Let us consider another chunking example. The nine items (Figure 5-1) are from a patient instruction on diabetes. If we attempt to commit them to memory in the original form, we face a tedious task of rote memorizing. However, if the nine items are chunked under three descriptive headings (Figure 5-2), they can be remembered more easily. Furthermore, the two important behavior items from the patient's point of view (what to do on sick days) now stand out from the other items and are more likely to be noticed and remembered.

- What ketones are
- Why ketones are produced
- What happens when ketones are produced
- Why test for ketones
- When to test for ketones
- How to test for ketones
- What ketone tests are available
- When to call the doctor
- What to do during sick days

FIGURE 5-1

Nine-item list from a diabetes instruction

KETONES: WHAT ARE THEY?
- What ketone are
- Why ketone are produced
- What happens when ketone are produced

TESTING FOR KETONES
- Why test for ketones
- When to test for ketones
- How to test for ketones
- What ketone tests are available

WHAT TO DO DURING SICK DAYS
- When to call the doctor
- What to do during sick days

FIGURE 5-2

Nine-item list "chunked" under three subheadings

Short-term memory has a short retention time. This memory usually lasts from a few hundred milliseconds to less than a minute. In very unusual instances with some people, the memory may last up to about an hour if it is not "overwritten" by some other stimulus or additional information. For most practical purposes, it lasts less than a minute. The information must be moved into the long-term memory quickly if patients are to remember new information. Quick conversion into long-term memory is necessary even for health instructions in the more "permanent" media, such as written instructions.

Patients with low literacy skills read written health care materials word by word. The one-word-at-a-time reading method slows down the reading process. By the time they arrive at the end of a long sentence, they may have forgotten many of the preceding words. Thus, they may have read every word without knowing the meaning of the sentence.

For written instructions, one remedy for the word-at-a-time reading process is to write shorter sentences using more common words. Another way to speed up the mental processing of words is to use words consistently throughout your instruction. Stay with one well-understood term such as "your meals" rather than using a variety of words, such as "diet," "meal plan," "diet prescription." It takes too long to decode all the various terms, compare them, and reclassify them. Such a variety of words are likely to be lost or misunderstood. (More than one patient has understood "diet prescription" to be an add-on—like a drugstore prescription—and has eaten her diet prescription in addition to her regular meals.)

For a video instruction, a remedy is to provide time for the viewer to convert the new information to long-term memory before the time is up on the short-term memory. (Approaches to doing this for written materials are covered in Chapter 6, and for video in Chapter 8.)

Please return to the sample instruction you selected at the beginning of the chapter. Look for sentences longer than 15 words, especially those that contain one or more difficult words. If you found several, it is likely that, for low literacy patients, comprehension will suffer because the sentences take too long to read.

Getting into the long-term memory

The long-term memory lasts for days and years and has no practical limit in terms of capacity. The two key factors to get information "learned" by the long-term memory are **association** and **interaction**.

Associate the new information with what the patient already knows. We learn new information by tieing it to something we already know—a thing we know, an experience we've had, something we've felt, something we've seen, something we have smelled or tasted. Here are some ways to do this:

- Explain the new words by context and examples.
- Ask the patients to say what it reminds them of.
- Use several media: pictures, tactile actions, and demonstrations.
- Use a mnemonic—like the "A,B,C" to remember the three steps in CPR.
- Relate it to something comparable they can do at home.

To explain the amount of salt to add to infant oral rehydration solution for use in third world countries, an instruction tells the amount of salt and then says,"Be sure it is no saltier than tears."

Compared with words, pictures and illustrations help learning and recall because there are many more access points in the brain to use for their recall.[2] Indeed, a picture may be worth 1,000 words. How often have we recognized someone's face, but cannot recall the name; or we can just "see" a book, its size, color, and location on the shelf, but cannot recall the title or author?

Involve the patient via interaction. Educators have long known that students learn more rapidly when they interact with new information to be learned. This has been confirmed with physical evidence from recent neurophysical research, which shows that when a person interacts with new information, a chemical change takes place in the brain that fosters long-term memory of that information.[3] When we do not interact, the chemical change does not take place, or does so more weakly.

Here are some ways to build patient interaction into instructions:

- Ask the patient to tell you about the new information in his own words.
- Present a problem: "How/when will you do this when you go home?"
- Ask the patient what problems he has or expects to have to comply.
- Ask questions during a teaching/learning session; dialogue with the patient.
- For written materials, ask questions and leave blanks for patient write-in, or check-off, or ask the patient to circle a selected picture.
- For small group instruction, foster interaction between members of the group.

Rather than ask patients if they understand your instruction, ask them to tell you—in their own words—about the instruction. Ask them to tell you how they will carry out the instruction, and the kinds of problems they face to comply. *In their own words* is important because the test of comprehension is the conversion of information from one format to another. Examples of this conversion, in addition to converting your words into their words, are showing or demonstrating the action called for in the instruction.

Interaction can be built into instructions in any media. If it is written, include a question to be answered after every important topic. The reader must write something, or circle or check something, to respond. For audiotapes, include a few direct questions to the listener and include a pause to allow the patient to respond; then, after a pause, give the right answer. A single-page worksheet can be developed for use in patient interaction for audio- or videotaped instructions. If it is a demonstration, have the patient demonstrate back to you. Other interaction methods include the use of games, interactive television, and interactive multimedia instructions. These interactive methods are described in more detail in the following chapters.

At this point, close your eyes and say out loud the ways you can build interaction into your patient instructions.

To summarize, to get information into the patient's memory:

SHORT-TERM MEMORY

   – Gain the patient's attention.
   – Present no more than seven items at a time.
   – Get to the point without delay.

LONG-TERM MEMORY

   – Associate new information with what the patient already knows.
   – Involve the patient in interaction with the information.
   – Repeat or review.

Returning now to your pamphlet, is the new information presented in association with something the patient already knows? Are there opportunities for patient interaction? If you can say even a limited "yes" to both of these questions, the pamphlet goes a long way toward being an effective instruction.

The Role of Logic, Language, and Experience

We learn new information by adding it to what we already know in terms of our logic, our language, and our experience. Unless the logic, language, and experience inherent in the new information is a reasonable match with our logic, language, and experience, we are not inclined to accept it or learn it.[4] For example, for many people it is not logical to keep on taking medication when they feel well. Using this logic, it is entirely reasonable to stop taking medication for hypertension or tuberculosis when they begin to feel okay.

Language mismatches occur where unexplained and unfamiliar words are used in a health care instruction. Mismatches also occur where familiar words are used in unfamiliar contexts, for example, referring to blood glucose levels in the "normal range." Patients may think "that's not for me" and discard the advice given.

The concept of matching the logic, language, and experience of health instructions with the logic, language, and experience of the patients is shown graphically in Figure 5-3. If one of your patient instructions is not getting through to your patients, look for possible mismatches in logic, language, or experience.

FIGURE 5-3

Matching the instruction to the patient's logic, language, experience

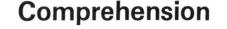

Comprehension

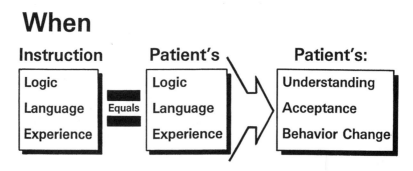

The Effect of Cultural Differences on Logic, Language, and Experience

Language

Language is the most "visible" of the cultural differences and is also one of the more easily managed factors. Under most circumstances oral and written instructions can be translated from English to any language. Multi-language books are available to aid in obtaining a medical history, and in many hospitals and clinics staff are available to translate for patients.[5]

Translation tips

What about translating pamphlets and handouts into other languages? The tendency is to translate the pamphlet directly from English into another language, and give it to the person to read. This is seldom a productive approach because of cultural differences and literacy limitations. The cultural "baggage" of the English version may be unsuitable for another culture, and many patients don't read well in any language. Before you take that step, ask an interpreter to talk with a sample of the intended population to determine if the instruction needs to be in that language or whether a simplified version in English, which includes lots of illustrations, could meet their needs just as well.

If you decide to translate material, have several (at least three) members from the culture work with you in the overall design and approach. Often graphics, diet lists, and procedures do not translate with the same meaning in other languages. Once the material is translated, have another person back-translate it into English to make sure that omissions or additions have not been made.

- Use a family member who speaks English as a translator, providing the person has sufficient fluency in English to communicate your messages.
- A number of community services are becoming available to meet specific translation needs. For example, some churches offer translation services; major metropolitan airport authorities and community refugee centers have translation help.

There are other ways to communicate when you don't speak the language:

- Use pictures, synthetic body models, and demonstrations with actual equipment to get your message across.
- Try simulation experiences—for example, using play equipment such as "Play Dentist"—to teach patients what to expect before having the procedure.
- Audiotapes made in the dialects of your patient population can be useful in presenting routine information, i.e., admission procedures, orientation to the facility, etc.
- Stories on audio cassettes appropriate to the culture can make both children and adults feel more at home.
- Drawing pictures has a high value in some cultures. Ask the patient to draw how he feels or what he understands about a health instruction.

Testing for comprehension using oral translation: After giving an instruction, ask the patient to show, draw, or communicate with gestures what he is supposed to do. Ask the patient to repeat the feedback if there is hesitation or his body language indicates uncertainty.

Experience

It is difficult for us to know and understand the experience factor of patients from other cultures. All of us interpret information through the filter of our experiences. And some of the most ordinary requests that we make in the health care system are not within the experiences of other cultures. For example:

Upon a return visit to a clinic a non-English-speaking patient had not made the progress expected. When asked if he needed a refill of his prescription, it turned out he had never had it filled in the first place. The prescription slip was still in the glove compartment of his car. He didn't know what to do with it.

In many cultures, tradition dictates how new information should be presented. Therefore, the organization as well as the sequence of information can change with the culture. These cultural variations may include giving a little information at a time; using stories to instruct; building on extended family networks; learning by rote (memorizing). These cultural variations are an additional factor to be considered for low literacy patients. A departure from their cultural tradition makes it harder for them to learn from it. In other words, it takes a different kind of presentation than a literal translation from English to their language. The following two examples illustrate this point.

When computers from the United States were introduced into Japan, the instructions were literally translated from English to Japanese. The literal translation didn't work. The Japanese prefer to be drawn into the material more gradually than American readers. American readers are accustomed to a brief introduction, followed by an overview of the product, and its functions, and then a step-by-step tutorial.

Japanese readers were uncomfortable seeing the big picture first; they prefer to be introduced to the parts one at a time before encountering the whole. But they want some precautions up front about the problems that might arise.[6]

This second example illustrates how the experience and customs of another culture led to a change in the focus of a health care instruction:

The Los Angeles Cancer Education Project conducted learner verification of a number of national and local publications with a group of potential users from the Hispanic community. The group found the materials unsuitable because they dealt with facts, rather than with people and their concerns. They felt keenly enough to create a new publication based on extended family experiences with cancer. Hablaremos Sobre Cancer Dentro de la Familia (Let's Talk About Cancer Among the Family) became the centerpiece for a comprehensive community effort to detect early cancer. Family participation for cancer detection is more culturally appropriate than individual participation.[7]

How do you learn about the experience factor? The best way is to work with a sample of your intended audience who are bilingual. Explain your purpose and what needs to be communicated. Ask for their advice on the best ways to present the information. And if possible, have them write it in the native language directly.

If you have no direct access to the population, network with several people in the community who have current access to your intended audience.[8] Ministers, priests, other religious leaders, school systems, community service agencies, and sometimes police agencies can be of assistance. In some communities minorities have formed their own business associations and they can be of considerable help.

Logic

The third component of comprehension in a cultural context is logic: what makes sense to you and me and what makes sense to people with other values and beliefs. In our culture it makes sense to educate the patient directly. Our assumption is that each person manages his own health care. But in other cultures the critical decision making is influenced by others, i.e., the godmother, the priest, the minister, or by an outside group such as a council of elders. In those instances, the target audience broadens to include not only the patient but also the significant decision makers.

For example, one of the authors was teaching breast self-examination in another culture. The women listened politely. They wondered about the wisdom of doing it, however, because if they found a lump, it would be a council of elders who would decide whether anything should be done about it.

In many other cultures it is logical for the authority figure to give "orders." Nobody asks questions. In fact, to ask questions because you didn't understand can be perceived as being critical of the authority figure. What does all this mean for patient education? Patients may need encouragement to ask questions. Pamphlets that model questions can be a great help to legitimatize and sanction asking them.

Patients need to be taught to expect medical personnel to ask questions, i.e., for a medical history. The perception "if he has to ask so many questions he can't be a very good doctor" needs to be reoriented. Patients must learn what to expect in a medical encounter. This is a key area for health education.

It is a common practice in the American culture to lighten up serious information with humor, using cartoons or caricature techniques. This practice can lead to misunderstandings. In many cultures humor is not used when dealing with serious health problems. The perception of non-English speakers may be that the information is not serious or "you don't care about me." Test any material of this type with the intended audience before using it.

Cultural Suitability: What Is Being Done

Health practitioners frequently ask, "How can we know what is appropriate and understandable for another culture?" This poses a challenge for health education programs in terms of both language and culture. One approach is to produce patient education instructions in all of the frequently used languages in the area. For example, the Department of Health in Hawaii now produces hepatitis pamphlets in Vietnamese, Laotian, and Cambodian languages; the Women, Infant Children's program (WIC) in Massachusetts translates infant feeding information into eight languages; bilingual pamphlets in Spanish/English are as common in Philadelphia as they are in Florida and California; a video on AIDS in Creole with English subtitles is used in the migrant health programs.

On the national scene, legislation to include minorities in health care research and service programs has provided an impetus to understand more about other cultures. This issue is being addressed in a number of ways: through national and regional conferences on multi-cultural communication methods; via new guidebooks on how to work with culturally diverse communities;[9] and through a computerized database of minority health-related resources at local, state, and national levels.[10]

An approach to achieve culturally appropriate materials is to use health practitioners who are members of that culture to develop the materials. During 1992 and 1993, the National Cancer Institute used this approach to develop nutrition materials for seven different cultures.[11]

When resources are limited, perhaps the most practical approach to cultural suitability is to ask the advice of members of the culture during the planning and development stages, and then use the learner verification and review (LVR) process described in Chapter 10 to assess suitability and to make any needed revisions.

Summary of methods to obtain cultural suitability of materials

1. Read the references on methods to develop culture suitable materials.
2. Obtain advice from members of the culture during the planning/development.
3. Produce materials in the languages of your patient population.
4. Use practitioner panels from the culture to develop health materials.
5. Assess the suitability of draft and finished material using the LVR process.

References

1. Miller GA (1956): The magical number seven. Psychology Review 63:81.
2. Jonassen DN (ed) (1982): The Technology of Text. Englewood Cliffs, NJ: Educational Technology Publications, pp. 91–120.
3. Thompson RF, Greenough W (November 1989): "Researchers gain insight into how brain remembers," Phoenix, AZ: Society for Neuroscience. Reported in Philadelphia Inquirer, Wed., Nov. 1, 1988, p.8.
4. Colvin RJ, Root JH (1972): Tutor: Techniques Used in the Teaching of Reading. Literacy Volunteers of America. Syracuse, NY, p. 49.
5. Carlin C (ed) (1989): Do You Understand? Communicating with the Non-English-Speaking Patient. Literacy Volunteers of America. Syracuse, NY.

6. Simply Stated (July 1985): Monthly newsletter of the Document Design Center. No. 57. Writing user manuals for Japanese readers, as contained in Journal of Reading 30(1): October 1986, ISSN 0022-4103, p. 13.

7. Curry, VM (1976): Mexican American Cancer Education Project. Los Angeles Co. Branch, Division of the American Cancer Society. Written for the Upjohn Health Education Project, Making Health Education Work, Washington, DC, American Public Health Association.

8. Office of Minority Health-Resource Center (Coordinates resource persons network to provide technical assistance), PO Box 37337, Washington, DC 20013-7337.

9. Randall-David, Elizabeth (1989): Strategies for Working with Culturally Diverse Communities and Clients. Association for the Care of Children's Health, 3615 Wisconsin Ave. NW, Washington, DC 20016. ISBN 0-937821-58-6. 96p.

10. Office of Minority Health Resource Center, PO Box 37337, Washington, DC 20013-7337, (301)-587-1938.

11. National Cancer Institute, Special Populations Branch (1992–1993): Nutrition Guidelines for Ethnic Groups. Washington, DC.

6

"My patients have a mix of literacy skills. Can one material satisfy all?"

Writing the Message

The health community is a "written culture": print materials are used extensively in all aspects of health care. Patients are expected to read and remember, to learn and comply with the advice presented. We see it as their responsibility.

Nurses and doctors have responsibilities too: to provide written materials that are easily understood, that are motivating, that help the patient to learn, and that are culturally suitable. How well are these responsibilities being lived up to?

The Mismatch Between Instructions and Patients

Although many written materials are suitable, most current materials have shortcomings that make them difficult to understand. The most serious shortcomings are:

- Too much information is included. This will discourage poor readers and will tend to obscure the priority information for all readers.
- Readability levels are too high for the average patient.
- The reader is not asked to interact with the material, so this opportunity for better learning and recall is lost.
- Difficult/uncommon words are seldom explained with examples.

What are the readability levels of current health education materials? From Figure 6-1, we see that the patient education materials have a wide range of readability levels, and that more than half the materials are too difficult for the average American adult.

The materials in Figure 6-1 were drawn from health instructions on a wide variety of topics and from many sources.[1] Does this mean we should discard all our on-the-shelf materials with reading levels above 10th grade? Such action is probably not necessary. Chapter 9, Tips On Teaching, presents ways to help patients understand at least the most important information contained in these materials.

The readability mismatch leads to another undesirable result—a reduction in motivation to comply with the instruction. When patients struggle to read and understand an instruction, they become discouraged and lose a sense of self-efficacy. They may feel that if it is so difficult to read, it is probably too difficult to do anyway, so why try?

Noncompliance with difficult instructions is not surprising, but is the converse true? Do easy-to-read materials increase compliance? Bradshaw, Ley, and Kincey provide convincing evidence that they do. Patients not only have a higher rate of compliance, but they remember better and make fewer mistakes.[2] Fredrickson (1994) describes the beneficial effects of easy-to-read health materials for people with higher literacy skills—even those with college degrees learned and remembered more from the simpler materials.[3] Simpler instructions help everyone.

The good news is that patients don't lack intelligence—nearly all of them can learn anything they need to know about their health care. The even better news is that nurses and doctors can learn fairly rapidly to improve written instructions so they are more suitable for their patients.

In this chapter you will find strategies to reduce the literacy and learning mismatches noted above, and ways to plan, write, and produce health care materials that work. We suggest strategies that would include the target audience—your patients—to help in your planning and writing tasks.

FIGURE 6-1

Readability levels of 1,234 health-care materials compared with the average reading skills of adult Americans. (*Source:* C. C. Doak, L. G. Doak, Patient Learning Associates, Potomac, MD)

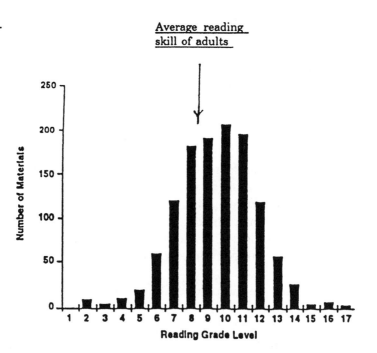

Other resources for clear writing: The literature is rich with advice on clear and simple writing. Flesch (1946) and Bailey (1984) suggest we should write the way we talk, and they offer other useful advice.[4,5] Duffy (1985) suggests ways to make text more usable to readers.[6] Doak (1985) applied these principles to patient education materials.[7] White (1988) and Jonassen (1982) offer advice on typography and layout to make text easier to read.[8,9] Wileman (1993) offers ways to make visuals more "readable."[10] And during the past few years a number of booklets and handbooks have been published on this subject by government agencies.[11,12] These authors offer useful advice and we draw upon them as well as other sources for the practical guidelines of clear writing offered in this chapter.

Simplifying Materials: The Planning Phase

A little planning makes the writing go easier. An hour or two spent in planning can save days or weeks later on. The planning steps you use will depend on your own circumstances and objectives, but we suggest you consider those shown in Chapter 2, Box 2-2, and those listed in Box 6-1 below.

Defining the audience

Defining the audience seems like such an obvious first step, but it is often overlooked. A few moments to consider the makeup of the target audience(s) can pay big dividends. For example, if you are writing a booklet on managing

BOX 6-1

Planning steps for written materials

DEFINE AND INVOLVE THE AUDIENCE

- Ages, genders, cultures
- Their literacy levels and readiness to learn
- Which learning theories apply?
- Include a few patients in the planning and writing phases

LIMIT THE OBJECTIVE(S) AND THE MESSAGE

- Decide on the minimum educational objective
- List topics that *must* be included

WRITING AND PRODUCTION PHASES

- Select format(s): description, story, Q & A, audio, video, etc.
- Decide how to include interaction
- Decide which words or phrases need explanatory examples and include them

QUALITY ASSURANCE

- Plan to test the draft and the final with a few patients/clients
- Use the checklist, readability test, SAM (Chapter 3)
- Document the assessment results

incontinence, you would write it at a lower readability level because this older audience has twice the functional illiteracy rate as the general population. Also, you would use larger type, perhaps 14 point, for easier reading. If writing about getting a pap smear or a mammogram for middle-aged women from specific countries or ethnic groups, you might consider including men among your expected audience for they may be the decision makers for these matters in the family.

Consider the learning and behavior theories that apply in your instructional situation. For example, the stage(s) of readiness to learn and comply is a key factor in selecting the content and approach for an instruction. If your audience may be in any stage of readiness (from creating awareness to maintaining a behavior) you may need to include topics suitable for all stages. (See Prochaska and DiClemente, 1985, Coping and Substance Abuse, Academic Press, New York, pp. 345–363.)

Involving the target audience in materials design

An ad hoc design assistance group or focus group made up of a few patients/clients can be of great help during the planning and writing phases.[13,14] Patients are almost always quite willing to serve as unpaid collaborators and can make valuable suggestions. For example, in preparing a new booklet on good nutrition for pregnant teenagers, nurses and nutritionists at the Philadelphia Health Department enlisted the aid of pregnant teens from three different cultures.[15] For healthy lunches (a topic in the draft booklet) teens were advised on healthy foods and how to prepare them. At an informal focus group meeting, the following dialogue ensued:

NURSE: And so we suggest you select baked or broiled foods, rather than fried.
TEENS: But we can't do that!
NURSE: Why not?
TEENS: Because we go to the food truck.
NURSE: The what?
TEENS: We buy lunch from the food trucks outside where we work.
NURSE: Oh.

The draft booklet was modified to explain how to make healthy lunch selections from a food truck, and to ask the food truck man to carry more healthy baked or broiled foods and more fruits and salads.

When working with a focus group, provide samples of possible choices and get the opinion of the group to guide your selection. What you ask in the interview session is influenced by what you wish to find out. Listen carefully. Listen more than you talk. Listen for their vocabulary. If they say "shots" instead of "immunizations" or "injections," perhaps their word should be used in the instruction. Take notes, have someone else take notes, or tape the discussion. You are not obliged to heed the advice you get, only to consider it. An hour spent this way can stimulate your own ideas and boost your project considerably.

In lieu of a focus group, individuals from the target audience can help. Writers have used individuals from WIC groups or Head Start parents to help. A health educator in Boston enlisted the help of prostitutes to select the most appropriate words in an AIDS pamphlet intended for them.[16] In addition to wording, the target audience can aid in the suitability of illustrations and content.

Some nurses have enlisted the aid of hospital patients, one at a time. Patients are pleased to be asked their opinions, and the comments from even one or two patients can offer valuable insights.

Limiting the objective(s)

Limiting and defining the learning objective(s) are sometimes the hardest parts of the writing process. The objective may be defined by first doing a needs assessment. Another approach is to ask, "What effect or outcome do I want for the patients? What are patients to *do* with the instruction?" Are they to learn to perform a new procedure? Is the objective to strengthen an attitude; to move the person to seek help or advice; to provide new information to ease a worry? The answers to these questions can help to define the core concept (that is, the theme or main idea). An example of a limited objective for a hypertension instruction is shown in Table 6-1.[17]

Notice that a number of other possible topics are *not* included in Table 6-1, for example, reduced weight, cutting down on salt, getting more exercise, regular physical exams. These topics, although important, are not consistent with the stated objectives. They would be covered in separate instructions. Several short instructions that are easy to digest are almost always better than one larger instruction that looks difficult simply because of its size.

You may want to stop at this point and take a look at a current health care pamphlet or booklet used in your health care setting. What appears to be the objective or core concept for the reader? How much of the information in the pamphlet could be cut out and still meet the objective? It is more difficult for patients to remember large amounts of information. Solid pages of print are a turnoff for most of us—and for those who have trouble reading they are a *stop sign.* So we need to start with this question:

TABLE 6-1
Example: Limited education objectives for a hypertension instruction

OBJECTIVES (FOR PATIENT)	"MUST INCLUDE" TOPICS	INTERACTIVE QUESTIONS
1. Understand what hypertension is	What is hypertension and what is patient's blood pressure?	What is high blood pressure? What is your blood pressure (HBP)?
2. Follows medication regimen	Dangers of hypertension	What are some dangers *to you* from HBP?
	Taking medicine can control hypertension	How can you lower your blood pressure?
	Must take medication every day even if you feel okay	What about taking medication on days you feel okay?

"What is the least I can include to give the reader the information and motivation needed to change behavior or perform the procedure?"

Before presenting the guidelines for writing, you may want to refer back to the five guidelines for health instruction material in Box 2-2, Chapter 2. We will assume you have done this and, if you are preparing to write an instruction, you have already limited your objective to the core concept you want to present, and have defined the key information your instruction must contain to meet that objective.

Guidelines for Writing

The practical guidelines shown below are the essence of the best the authors have found in the literature. The guidelines are few in number and, with a little practice, are easy to apply.

1. **Write the way you talk; use active voice.**
2. **Use common words, and, on average, use short sentences.**
3. **Give examples to explain hard words.**
4. **Include interaction and reviews.**

Bailey (1984) tells us to "write the way you talk."[18] If you do this, three beneficial things happen to the written material:

1. *It is easier to read.* The readability level automatically drops several grades–often five or six grade levels.
2. *It becomes more interesting to read.* Your patients will *want* to read it.
3. *It is easier to understand.* The extra words we use when we talk—the redundant or amplifying words—give the reader additional paths to understand the message.

Perhaps the best way to write the way you talk is to imagine that you are facing a patient and telling him or her your message. Say it out loud and write down exactly what you've said. Don't worry about grammatical accuracy; this is just a draft you can revise later.

When you write as though you are talking to a member of your target audience, your writing will have a more personal and friendly tone and it can be just as accurate as more formal writing. Consider the two AIDS instructions shown in Box 6-2, one written formally, the other written simply.

Active voice

When the subject of the sentence is the doer, you have active voice, and that's easier to read. A message written in active voice is more likely to move the reader to action than the same message in passive voice. Passive voice is signaled by the verb *to be* and usually by the word *by*, and you will often find a helping verb included too. Examples of sentences in active and passive voice are shown in Box 6-3.

<table>
<tr><td>**BOX 6-2**

A comparison: formal vs.
simple writing</td><td>FORMAL WRITING
(AIDS INSTRUCTION)

Sometimes the preliminary test results are positive when the person is not infected. A positive AIDS test should be reconfirmed by a different lab technique to assure that it is accurate.</td><td>SIMPLE WRITING
(AIDS INSTRUCTION)

If your AIDS test comes back positive, you may not have AIDS. Have the test done again using another method. Sometimes the first lab test gives a false reading.</td></tr>
</table>

<table>
<tr><td>**BOX 6-3**

A comparison: active vs.
passive voice</td><td>ACTIVE VOICE: (BETTER)

Take your medicine with your meals.

Warn patients about side effects.

The nurse will bandage your arm.</td><td>PASSIVE VOICE: (NOT AS GOOD)

Medicine should be taken at mealtimes.

Patients should be warned about side effects.

Your arm will be bandaged by the nurse.</td></tr>
</table>

Use common words

Which words are common and are understood by nearly all patients? The words you would use in talking with a nontechnical friend tend to be more common than words you would write. Another way to assess how common a word may be is to look it up in the *Word Frequency Book* to see where it ranks among 86,000 English words.[19] Words that rank among the first 3,000 are common words.

Short words tend to be more common and are preferred, for example *doctor* vs. *physician*. However, three classes of words that may seem very common are problems because they may mean different things to different patients. These are words that represent *concepts* and *categories*, and express *value judgments*.

Concept words describe a general idea or an abstract framework or reference, and are often misunderstood. Diabetics are instructed to eat a "variety" of foods, and to keep "in balance." Another example: the patient who reads "Keep your glucose level within a normal range" may know the meaning of normal, and that she has a range in her kitchen. To make such concept words understood by patients, include an example immediately after using them. In the latter example you might include, "This means to keep your blood sugar somewhere between 70 and 120; that is the range of sugar numbers that means your blood sugar is normal—that it's okay."

Category words describe groups of things, such as the categories of products listed in the Yellow Pages of the telephone book. Many people with low literacy skills can't use the Yellow Pages because they don't understand the category words. For example, if they want to rent a house, they won't find it under "house," but under "real estate–residential–rental." The problem with unexplained category words is illustrated in the following learner verification dialogue between a health educator and Fred, a kidney dialysis patient. The patient has just read a paragraph telling him to eat red meat, and to avoid eating shell fish and poultry.

EDUC: Fred, you've just read this page. Could you tell me what it is all about?
FRED: It's about the kind of meat I'm supposed to eat.
EDUC: You've got the idea. What kinds of meat do you eat for supper?
FRED: Oh, steak or fried chicken.
EDUC: Do you eat chicken often, or only once in a while?
FRED: Oh, all the time. I like fried chicken.
EDUC: What about poultry?
FRED: I never eat poultry; we're not supposed to have that!

Value judgment words often describe amounts or thresholds for action. Here are some examples (italicized):

One post-op. instruction reads, "If you have *excessive* bleeding, call your doctor." How much blood is excessive? The nurse and doctor know, but chances are the patient does not.
Exercise *regularly*; don't lift anything *heavy*; get *adequate* rest.

You can resolve these problems by using more specific words rather than value judgment words, or by explaining what is meant by the value judgment word. For example, "adequate rest" might be explained: "For the next week you need a lot of rest and that means at least 8 hours of sleep each night and a 2-hour rest period lying down each afternoon."

Short sentences

In general, short sentences are easier to read and understand compared to long sentences. A good rule is to keep sentence length under 15 words; under 10 is even better. But there are exceptions. Sentences should be kept short, but not at the expense of conversational style. If it is more natural to express some parts of the message in a sentence that is longer, write it that way. The redundant words and natural flow of the language will make it easier to understand.

Give examples to explain uncommon words

In addition to concept, category, and value judgment words, many words used in health care settings are uncommon and need an example if they are to be understood. For the reader, the example may call to mind a mental image so the meaning of the word is perceived and more easily remembered. For example, "As the prostate continues to grow, it can squeeze the urethra—like pinching a straw—and interfere with the normal flow of urine." The words "pinching a straw" provide the example and may create a mental image.

Examples also lighten up the text and make it more interesting to read. One of the most frequent comments by reviewers of the manuscript for this book was that they liked the many examples given.

Include interaction

Perhaps more than anything else, interaction can make instructions easier to learn and remember. And it is one of the least used features in health instruction. An analysis by the authors of 100 materials revealed that only one out of five included any interaction with the reader. Some ways to include interaction are:

1. Write a short question and leave a blank line for the patient to write in the answer.
2. Ask the reader to circle one among several pictures to make the right choices.
3. Pose a problem, and ask patients to write or say out loud how it can be resolved. Or ask the patient to demonstrate what was read.
4. Ask a few questions verbally after a patient has read the material.
5. Ask a group of patients a question and let them discuss their answers.

An example of how interaction can be included in written material is shown in Figure 6-2.[20]

FIGURE 6-2

Interaction and review are included via questions to be answered

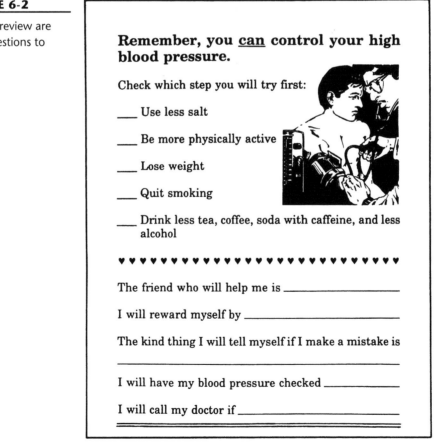

Remember, you <u>can</u> control your high blood pressure.

Check which step you will try first:

___ Use less salt

___ Be more physically active

___ Lose weight

___ Quit smoking

___ Drink less tea, coffee, soda with caffeine, and less alcohol

♥ ♥

The friend who will help me is _____

I will reward myself by _____

The kind thing I will tell myself if I make a mistake is

_____

I will have my blood pressure checked _____

I will call my doctor if _____

Writing models

You may be wondering, "Which information should I present first? What should be the sequence?" Depending on your purpose for the patient, the answer can be found in one or a combination of models as shown in Table 6-2.

As noted in Chapter 2, the sequence of information based on the health belief model is (1) you are at risk, (2) but there is something you can do about it, and (3) you will get personal benefits if you do. An example instruction based on the health belief model is shown below.

"You are in the high-risk group for cancer. But you can cut your chances of getting cancer if you'll do just three things: (1) quit smoking now, (2) eat less red meat, and (3) eat more fruits and vegetables.

Take a smoking cessation class, and get "the patch" to help you quit smoking. Instead of steaks and roast beef, eat fish or pasta, and add fruit to every meal. Eat red meat only once a week. You can do this. Your spouse will help you.

If you do these three things now, you'll have a much better chance to live to see your grandkids grow up, and you will feel better and look younger."

The story model builds empathy and interest by engaging the reader's emotions and feelings in the message. Story models usually involve some controversy or tension to build interest. Stories can also have powerful cultural attractiveness and may be the natural way that information is transmitted in that culture. A dialogue with or without pictures carries the story and holds attention via the "power of the overheard conversation."[21] One form of the story model is the adult comic strip or photo-novella. This format is illustrated in Chapter 7, Figure 7-19.

The medical model is the least suitable of all the models for patient instructions. Both the content and the sequence of information are in conflict with what most patients need to know and want to know. This sequence of information is more suited to subject instructions for health practitioners. The medical model sequence is usually presented as follows: (1) description of the disease, its history, and the disease process; (2) statistics on its frequency, cure rate, etc.; (3) various forms of treatment; (4) the efficacy of the treatments and

TABLE 6-2
Writing models and their purposes

WRITING MODEL	PURPOSE OR OBJECTIVE OF THE INSTRUCTION
1. Health belief model	To change a patient's behavior(s) and attitude
2. Procedural model	To present a series of steps that must be done in a specified sequence
3. Story model	When raising empathy and interest is needed to gain attention and acceptance
4. Newspaper model	Most important part is given first; next parts are in order of descending importance; helpful for poor readers
5. Medical model	To teach health-care personnel, and for the few patients who want medical details

medications; (5) side effects; (6) other information. The medical model is described here so you will recognize it *and avoid using it for patient instructions.*

Additional Ways to Make Text Easy to Read

Use headers to group items together under a common headline. These captions are sometimes called advance organizers because they organize our thinking to anticipate the content of the text that is coming next. Poor readers don't organize well as they read. Groupings make it easier to remember. The best headers are those that express a complete thought or idea. These are better than one-word headers. (See Chapter 5, Figures 5-1 and 5-2, for examples of headers used for chunking.)

Place the key behavior information first, in the most powerful position. Just as first impressions often stick when we meet others, so too, the first part of the message is remembered best. The last part is a close second in importance. We often experience this when we can say the first or last line in a poem or a song, but can't remember the rest of the words.

Use the favored, up-front position for the core of your message—put the most important information or behavior in the position most likely to be remembered in your pamphlet or instruction.

When writing a sentence or paragraph, **give the context first,** before presenting new information. Doing this provides a place—a framework—for new information to fit before it arrives. When the context is given last, we must carry all the information along in our short-term memory. We must try to remember it all until we get to the end of the sentence or paragraph or list. Examples of context given first and last are shown in Box 6-4. In both examples the context words are in italics.

Typography and Layout

The type style and layout can create a user-friendly appearance so that patients want to read the material. Poor choices of type style and layout can

BOX 6-4	CONTEXT FIRST (EASY TO GRASP)	CONTEXT LAST (HARD TO GRASP)
A comparison: Context first vs. context last	*You can lower the amount of cholesterol in your body* by reducing animal food products and substituting low-fat or nonfat for whole diary products and increasing dietary fiber.	Reducing animal food products and substituting low-fat or nonfat for whole dairy products and increasing dietary fiber *can lower the amount of cholesterol in your body.*

do just the opposite. White (1988; see reference 8) offers extensive advice and many examples on how to achieve the former. The guidelines in Box 6-5 on the following page summarize how this can be done. Figure 6-3 on the following page shows a good example of the application of the guidelines.

Following is a sample of type fonts from the easiest to the hardest to read for readers at all skill levels, and samples of several type sizes.

Easy to read
- Serif Font (serifs are the little bars on the bottoms and tops of the letters)
- Sans-Serif Font

Hard to read
- ALL CAPITALS— NOTE THE RECTANGULARITY OF THE PRINT.
- *Italics and handwriting are difficult to read.*

This is 10-point type—more difficult to read.

This is 12-point type—much easier to read.

This is 13-point type—the best size for many materials.

TEXT WITH ALL CAPITALS IS DIFFICULT FOR READERS AT ALL SKILL LEVELS. Since all words are rectangular in shape, the reading cues provided by word shapes are lost. For example, notice the difference in the shapes of the word TRY and try—one can read the lowercase word almost by its shape alone. It is not necessary to read each letter.

One layout feature that can greatly increase a patient's perception of the importance of a booklet or pamphlet and takes less than a minute to do: Include a line for the patient's name on the cover. Some clinics that have done this have found that patients bring their booklets/pamphlets back with them on return visits, where before many had discarded the pamphlets.

Special Problems

Some written materials used in health care present special problems for patients with low literacy skills and often for high literacy patients as well. These materials are: (1) consent forms, (2) questionnaires, (3) lists and graphs. (Lists and graphs are discussed in Chapter 7, Visuals and How to Use Them.)

Consent forms: methods to simplify

Meade (1992) describes the reading difficulty and other problems with most consent forms used in health care.[22] The average readability of 44 consent forms was found to be at the mid-college level—hardly understandable by the average patient. Meade points out that making consent forms understandable is a responsibility shared by nurses because of their roles in patient care and research projects.

BOX 6-5

Guidelines for typography and layout

1. TYPE STYLE AND SIZE

- Use serif type and lowercase lettering, except where grammatically necessary to use capital letters.
- Use 12-point type or larger. (see example of type sizes).
- Do *not* use large or stylized initial letters (the big, fancy letters sometimes put at the start of a booklet or chapter).
- In general, do *not* use reverse print, that is, white on black.

2. LINE LENGTH

- Try to limit line length to 30 to 50 characters and spaces.
- Make the left edge of lines rectified (that is, all in a line).
- Leave right ends of lines ragged.

3. LAYOUT OF TEXT ON THE PAGE

- Leave some white space on the page to avoid a look of solid text.
- Use headers ("road signs") underlined or in bold print to introduce each new topic and to break up the appearance of a page of solid text.
- Use an eye-catcher—a box or larger font or an indent—to draw readers' eyes to the most important information.

FIGURE 6-3

A user-friendly layout that follows many of the guidelines (*Source:* Health Literacy Project, Health Promotion Council of Southeastern Pennsylvania, Philadelphia)

Where to go ?
The Emergency or the Clinic?

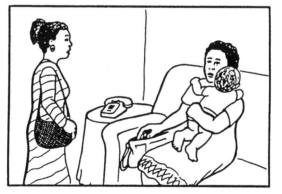

Frances: What is wrong with the baby?

Shirley: She is sick. Her nose is running and she has been crying a lot.

Frances: Yes, her head feels a little warm, too. Maybe she has a fever.

Shirley: Well, I am taking her to the Emergency.

Frances: I think you should take her to the clinic, not to the Emergency.

One way to find common words to replace difficult ones is to ask the lawyer or consent form writer for the meanings of difficult words in plain language. Write down their verbal responses and make the changes. For example, Meade presents the following comparative word list:

ORIGINAL WORDS	SIMPLER WORDS
chemotherapeutic agent	anticancer drug
determine	find out (or see if)
difficulties	problems
participate	take part
venipuncture	draw blood
intradermally	given under the skin

Consent forms are often written by highly trained medical staff and may then be modified by lawyers. The lawyers tend to include the long sentences and difficult words found in the law. However, this is not necessary. The legal demands and the literacy demands are not incompatible. A draft of a simplified living will consent form is shown in Figure 6-4. The original tested at the college level. The simplified version in Figure 6-4 is at about the 4th-grade level.

Questionnaires

Questionnaires present special problems for low literacy patients because (1) the purpose of the questionnaire is often not understood, (2) the readability level is often too high, (3) multiple formats are often employed for the answers, (4) they are too long. These problems can lead patients to guess at the answer. The result may be incomplete and confusing data, or no data at all. For example, a questionnaire mailed out to homeowners who did not request disaster relief aid (and to find out why not) was written at about the freshman college level. Very few responses were received.

Mayo and Rose (1991) report on research to develop a questionnaire to help screen out possible HIV (human immunodeficiency virus)–positive blood donors.[23] They found that the most reliable format for the questionnaire was a combination of pictures and short questions. Subsequent research for a questionnaire suitable for all blood donors, including those with low literacy skills, led to the development and testing of an interactive computer-based method to quickly obtain the information needed.

To make questionnaires acceptable and easier to understand, explain the purpose of the questionnaire in simple language. Give an example of the purpose. You may find it helpful to include a testimonial or supplemental explanatory material, possibly in the form of a set of pictures, a short video, or a verbal explanation.

Questionnaires are often developed by committees, and it shows. One difficult-to-understand questionnaire contained six different formats to answer the questions. Formats included were true/false, write in an answer, check a box, select a number from four possible answers, place an "X" on a continuum line, and darken a dot next to the chosen answer. Instead, use only one format for all questions, and show an example of how to answer and

FIGURE 6-4

An easy-to-read living will consent form (*Source:* Dr. Jane Root, Falmouth, Maine)

LIVING WILL
(Attorney Review Required)

To my doctor:

There may come a time when I can no longer tell you what I want. I may have no awareness and my mind may no longer work so that I know who I am or where I am. I may be near death and have no chance of recovery. Special equipment might be used to keep me alive a little while but it cannot bring back my health. If this is the case, I want you to take the following action:

(Sign only where you want your doctor to *take* the action.)

1. Use whatever you need to control pain.

    Signature: _____ Date: _____

2. *Do not* try to restart my heart or breathing if they should stop.

    Signature: _____ Date: _____

3. *Do not* use a respirator to keep me breathing.

    Signature: _____ Date: _____

4. *Do not* give me food and water through a tube.

    Signature: _____ Date: _____

Your signature: _____ Date: _____

Print or type your name: _____

••

This form was signed willingly while I watched:

Witness #1: _____ Witness #2: _____

Address: _____ Address: _____

Notary Public Statement
(for states which require this)

If you plan to travel, you should have this notarized.

You *must* give your doctor or other health provider a copy of this form to be sure your wishes are followed.

List here the names and addresses of those to whom you gave copies.
Name   Address

_____   _____
_____   _____
_____   _____
_____   _____

Remember: You can stop or chage this notice at any time. If you *do* change this notice, be sure to tell your doctor or other health provider.

mark the response. If a second answer format must be used, separate the questions by format, and tell the reader that you are changing the format for the answers and how to respond.

Patients with low literacy skills lose patience with long questionnaires, and may not complete them, or may just mark the answers at random. Experience has probably taught them that all they need to do to satisfy the request is to turn in a completed questionnaire. To prevent this from happening, keep the questionnaire short by asking only for the information that you definitely plan to use immediately or in the near future.

Summary

Think of the subject for a new health care instruction you may soon be writing. Then think how you will apply each of the points given in the summary below when you write the instruction.

PLANNING STEPS

- Define and involve the target audience.
- Limit the objectives and the message.
- Decide on message format, interaction, and examples.
- Plan to test for quality assurance.

WRITING THE MESSAGE

- Write the way you talk; use active voice.
- Use common words and short sentences.
- Give examples to explain uncommon, concept, category, and value judgment words.
- Include interaction and review.

References

1. Doak C, Doak L (November 10, 1992): Health Communication Strategies That Work. Presented at the American Public Health Association annual conference, Washington, DC.
2. Bradshaw P, Ley P, Kincey J (1975): Recall of medical advice: Comprehensibility and specificity. Br J Soc Clin Psychol 14:55–62.
3. Fredrickson D (1994): Study of parent comprehension comparing a short polio vaccine information pamphlet containing graphics and simple language with the currently available Public Health Service brochure. Pediatrics, in press.
4. Flesch R (1946): The Art of Plain Talk; (1949): The Art of Readable Writing. New York: Harper and Row.
5. Bailey EP Jr (1984): Writing Clearly: A Contemporary Approach. Columbus, OH: CE Merrill.
6. Duffy TM, Waller R (1985): Designing Usable Texts. Orlando, FL: Academic Press.
7. Doak CC, Doak LG, Root JH (1985): Teaching Patients with Low Literacy Skills. Philadelphia, PA: Lippincott.
8. White JV (1988): Graphic Design for the Electronic Age. New York: Watson–Guptill.
9. Jonassen DH (1982): The Technology of Text. Englewood Cliffs, NJ: Educational Technology Publications.
10. Wileman RE (1993): Visual Communicating. Englewood Cliffs, NJ: Educational Technology Publications.

11. U.S. Department of Health and Human Services, National Institutes of Health (NIH), National Cancer Institute (April 1992): Making Health Communications Programs Work: A Planner's Guide. NIH Pub. 92–1493.

12. Matiella AC, Middleton A, Thacker K (1991): Guidebook to Effective Materials Development for Health Education. Sacramento, CA: Tobacco Education Clearinghouse of California, Department of Health Services.

13. Debus M (1988): Handbook for Excellence in Focus Group Research. Academy for Educational Development, 1255 23rd St. NW, Washington, DC 20037.

14. Basch CE (1987): Focus group interview: an underutilized research technique for improving theory and practice in health education. Health Education Quarterly 14(4):411–448.

15. Scharf M, King E (1989): Healthy Foods Healthy Baby. Maternal and Infant Health, Philadelphia Department of Public Health, 500 South Broad St., Philadelphia, PA 19146.

16. Copan L (1993): AIDS pamphlet. AIDS Action Committee of Massachusetts, 131 Clarendon St., Boston, MA.

17. Working Group to Define Critical Patient Behaviors in High Blood Pressure Control (1979): JAMA 241(23):2534–2537.

18. Bailey EP, Jr. (1984) Writing Clearly: A Contemporary Approach. Charles E. Merrill Pub. Co., Columbus, OH 43216, p. 60.

19. Carroll JB, Davies P, Richman B (1970): Word Frequency Book. New York: Houghton Mifflin Co., American Heritage Publishing Co.

20. You Can Control Your High Blood Pressure (1994): Healthy Heart Program, Bangor, ME.

21. Walster E, Festinger L (1962): The effectiveness of "overheard" persuasive conversations. J Abnormal Psychol 65(6):395–402.

22. Meade CD, Howser DM (1992): Consent forms: how to determine and improve their readability. Oncology Nursing Forum 19(10):1523–1528.

23. Mayo DJ, Rose AM, et al. (June 1991): Screening potential blood donors at risk for human immunodeficiency virus. J Transfusion 30(5):466–474.

"What are the do's and don'ts in using visuals?"

Visuals and How to Use Them

Confucius was right when he said that a picture is worth a thousand words. Visuals enhance communication for everyone.[1] For poor readers the significance of visuals is even greater. This may be the only way that they can "read" and understand the health message.

This chapter points out the special needs of poor readers, and provides guidance to make visuals responsive to those needs. Your patients will obtain the full benefit from the visuals used in your instructions if you follow these guidelines.

This chapter is organized in three parts:

- Part 1: Rationale for Using Visuals and the Special Needs of Poor Readers
- Part 2: How to Select, Design, and Use Visuals Effectively
- Part 3: Making Lists and Graphics Understandable

Part 1: Rationale for Using Visuals and the Special Needs of Poor Readers

Visual presentations have been shown to be 43 percent more persuasive than unaided presentations.[2] The research on visuals and graphics shows that the memory systems in the brain favor visual storage, so when a message is visualized we remember it better than if we just read it or hear it.[3,4,5]

All of us learn through the five senses: seeing, hearing, touching, tasting, and smelling. Our learning styles are based on these sensory modes. We tend to use one learning style more than another, and for many people, visuals are a preferred style. Especially important for health education reasons, complex concepts can be understood easier through visual presentations. Our emotions are easily stimulated through the visual sense, so we respond quickly to what we see. The use of visuals in developing countries provides a rich resource to draw upon for practical examples of their value in health education.[6-11]

Unique characteristics of visuals for learning

Memory system factors: Everybody understands and remembers better when they *see* the message. The brain has more access routes and greater storage capacity for pictorial images than for words.[12] Therefore, details that might otherwise be lost can be reconstructed through visual association.

You can recognize these factors based on your own experiences. For example, do you remember saying, "I remember what the house looks like, and that it was next door to a church, but I've forgotten the name of the street." Although names and words may not be remembered, you can access enough of the image to reconstruct the picture.

Learning style preferences: Do you prefer to learn from pictures? Many people do. Some people have a visual learning style, so they need to see information as a way to understand it. The more vivid and real the visual impression of what is to be learned, the more likely it will be remembered.[13] Visuals make information vivid and real. Most poor readers rely on visuals and the spoken word. They try to get the sense of the instruction without having to struggle with text.

Complex concepts: Visuals can show a step-by-step procedure and make an entire action sequence seem easier to learn than explanations by text. The visuals can be logically grouped so that they become a memory set for easier recall.

Emotional impact: Visuals carry memorable emotional messages far surpassing words. In Figure 7-1, compare the emotional impact of the visual with that of the same message in text.

Another part of the rationale for using visuals is the fact that public expectations about information have changed. People expect to have their health messages visualized; the importance and value of the message is often equated with the quality of the production.

Special needs of poor readers

To understand the special needs of poor readers, it is helpful to first review the reading process that applies to all of us. What are the steps we all go through when we read visuals? They are:[14]

- Deciding to read or look (selective exposure)
- Finding the message
- Locating relevant details
- Interpreting the information (selective perception)
- Deciding to remember (or forget) the message (selective retention)

FIGURE 7-1

The meaning of the words become more powerful and clear when translated into the picture. (*Source:* Know the Facts About Fetal Alcohol Syndrome. Native American Community Board, PO Box 572, Lake Andes, SD 57356)

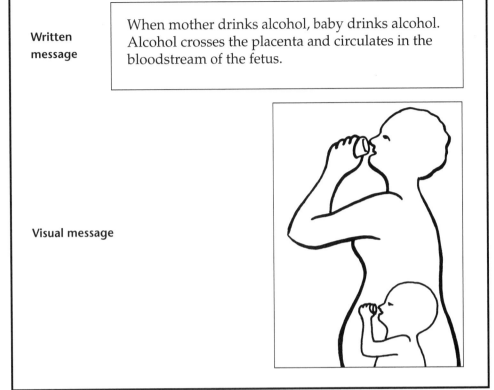

Written message

When mother drinks alcohol, baby drinks alcohol. Alcohol crosses the placenta and circulates in the bloodstream of the fetus.

Visual message

TABLE 7-1

Comparison of reading habits of visuals by skilled and poor readers

SKILLED READERS	POOR READERS
Systematically scan the visual to find the central concept	Eyes wander about page without finding the central focus of the visual
Quickly identify principal features	Skip over principal features
Separate key points from details	Eyes may focus on a detail
Quickly interpret information to arrive at meaning	Slow to interpret perceptual information; interpret words literally

With these steps in the process of reading visuals as a guide, it is possible to gain insight on the special needs of poor readers. Table 7-1 compares the reading habits of skilled and poor readers by using data from research on eye movements during reading.[15] The data point out why you need to think differently about visuals for poor readers.

The special needs of poor readers are revealed in the following ways. They often miss the purpose of the visual due to their random eye movements and their lack of attention to detail on principal features. The logic and experience expressed by the visual are often a mismatch for the poor reader. This mismatch makes it harder to get the meaning of the visual. If the poor readers cannot figure out the message quickly, they lose interest. For poor readers, not understanding an instruction is a common happening: the person feels that it's just not worth the effort.

Visuals are important and vital to communicate health messages to poor readers. However, not every kind of visual will be effective. The visuals must take into account the special needs of poor readers noted below.

The rest of the chapter discusses and illustrates visuals, lists, and graphs that are directed to meeting the special needs of poor readers.

Part 2: How to Select, Design, and Use Visuals Effectively

Once you have a clear educational objective written out, ask yourself: Can I reduce the amount of text and keep the reader interested by using visuals? Will visuals keep attention focused on the key points? Will a picture story be more likely to motivate the readers? Will visuals help simplify the steps in this instruction?

When you do this planning early in the idea or design stage, you will have a better outcome than if you wait until the draft is completed. To use visuals to meet the needs of poor readers:

1. Concentrate on main message.
2. Reduce the amount of reading in the text.
3. Provide visual cues and interaction.
4. Provide motivation.

1. Concentrate on main message

Because of their scientific origin, many health instructions for patients still include the textbook explanations of the disease process. These explanations usually contain too much detail and rely on a scientific background for comprehension.

Instead, patients need simple, easy-to-understand visuals focused on what they need to do. Four ways to concentrate on the main message are offered.

a. Focus on action patients should take

When trying to teach complex concepts, ask yourself: How do I expect patients *to apply* this information? If you focus on the action that you want the patient to take, two good things happen: (1) you attract the patient's attention, and (2) the complex information is cut. Use the visuals to give a sense of realism by helping the patient *see the action recommended.* For example, many times you will find you don't need the etiology of the disease.[16,17,18] People are more likely to take action if they see that the action is reasonable and doable (see Chapter 2).

The next two examples illustrate these points using an instruction for AIDS. Figure 7-2 shows facts about the transmission of disease process and Figure 7-3 on the following page shows the application of the facts to human behavior. It is the application of the facts that are most suitable for poor readers.

A note of caution: Don't use child-like imagery to try to simplify complex concepts. For example, a visual in a diabetes instruction shows dump trucks in the bloodstream delivering sugar to body cells for energy. Understanding this type of metaphor demands skills in inference. These skills are beyond unskilled readers who interpret information literally. The message could be discarded also because "that's for kids."

FIGURE 7-2

Facts about AIDS transmission. (*Source:* U.S. Surgeon General's Report on AIDS, 1991)

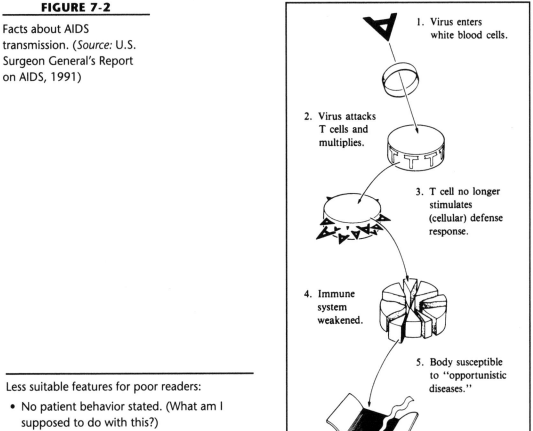

1. Virus enters white blood cells.

2. Virus attacks T cells and multiplies.

3. T cell no longer stimulates (cellular) defense response.

4. Immune system weakened.

5. Body susceptible to "opportunistic diseases."

Less suitable features for poor readers:

- No patient behavior stated. (What am I supposed to do with this?)
- Visuals are confusing.
- No emphasis on what's important.
- Language is difficult and hard to understand.

FIGURE 7-3

Behavior focus to prevent AIDS. Modeling behavior is more likely to motivate than presenting facts. (*Source:* Family Planning Association of Maine, ME AHEC, 1992)

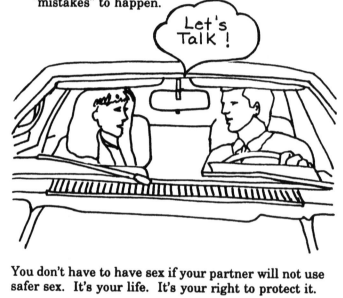

Plan ahead for safer sex.

1. Talk about sex. Tell your partner what you would like.

2. Practice what you will say. It's not easy to talk about sex.

3. Practice using a condom before you <u>need</u> to use one. A woman can unroll a condom onto a cucumber, a man onto his penis.

4. Keep condoms handy.

5. Don't drink and then have sex. Alcohol may cause "mistakes" to happen.

You don't have to have sex if your partner will not use safer sex. It's your life. It's your right to protect it.

More suitable features for poor readers:
- Reader can identify with the visual.
- The behavior action is clear.
- The language is easy to understand
- Familiar setting helps reader identification.

b. Present behavior (action to be taken) in bite-size steps

Partitioning the action, task, or procedure by using several "bite-size" images makes it seem easier to do as illustrated in Figure 7-4. It also gives the patient the chance to experience a number of small successes in learning and understanding. The belief that you can do it is one of the greatest motivating forces for behavior change.[19] Poor readers often have a low self-image, so use visuals to build self-efficacy. An overload of information reduces self-efficacy because the reader believes he cannot apply it.

FIGURE 7-4

Bite-size pieces of nutrition information make the advice seem easy to follow. (*Source:* "Jackie and Rhonda," National Cancer Institute, Branch of Special Populations, Bethesda, MD, *in press*)

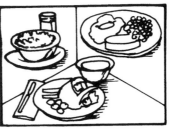

Eat three meals a day. Don't starve yourself and then stuff. It won't work.

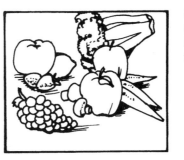

Throw away your grease can. Don't eat bacon grease and other meat fat.

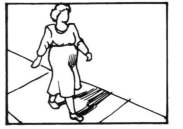

Cut down on the number of cakes and cookies you buy. Spend that money on fresh fruits and vegetables on sale.

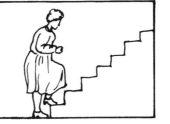

Take the stairs, and walk every time you can. It really helps to lose weight if you are more active.

Suitable features for poor readers:

- Pictures give an immediate image of what to do.
- One visual is presented for each "bite" of advice, making it seem easy to follow.
- Language is conversational.
- Familiar settings make reader feel comfortable.

Call a friend or take a walk instead of eating. Don't eat because you are bored, upset, or lonely.

c. Establish a familiar context to help understanding

Identification with the message is easier and quicker when the context in which it is presented seems familiar. Visuals can help establish the context of the familiar: they show people who look like they could be family or friends. The objects can be shown in ways to make them look familiar.

Figures 7-5 and 7-6 are a before-and-after comparison of unfamiliar context with familiar context: Figure 7-5 uses computer graphics clip art to show different types of chemical containers. The computer graphics did not work as a way of illustrating key concepts. When the staff tested the graphics with focus groups, they were found to be "cold" and unclear.

FIGURE 7-5

Stylized images of containers for hazardous materials. (*Source:* The Right to Understand: Linking Literacy to Health and Safety Training. Labor Occupational Health Program. University of California at Berkeley, 1994.)

Original version: Unfamiliar context

Less suitable for poor readers.

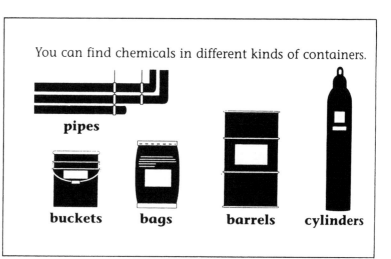

You can find chemicals in different kinds of containers.

pipes

buckets   bags   barrels   cylinders

FIGURE 7-6

Familiar images of containers for hazardous materials. (*Source:* The Right to Understand: Linking Literacy to Health and Safety Training. Labor Occupational Health Program. University of California at Berkeley, 1994.)

Familiar context: Revised version

Highly suitable for poor readers.

Do you work with chemicals found in:

☐ pipes

☐ bags   ☐ buckets   ☐ barrels   ☐ cylinders?

Chemicals can even be in the water, or in the ground.

For example, workers pointed out that the illustrations of containers were not shown in a workplace setting. Some of them thought the computer graphic used to illustrate a hazardous waste container was a keg of beer. These comments made it clear that some of the illustrations did not help explain the text.

In the revised version, Figure 7-6, the simple line drawings replace the computer graphics. The redrawn illustrations feature the same containers. However, they have been drawn as you might find them in the workplace. It's familiar.

A note of caution: Many readers place more trust in instructions that show people and settings with which they're familiar. Visuals can communicate a definite lifestyle. For instance, some instructions about good nutrition and exercise present the following images that are unsuitable for many people:

- Pictures of a carrot in a briefcase or dried fruit in a desk will lose credibility with many blue-collar workers.
- Pictures of golf clubs and sailing boats as examples of exercise are a mismatch with the lifestyle of many readers.
- Hairdos, facial characteristics, and jewelry or clothing styles unlike those of the reader might not work.

If one pamphlet is going to serve a variety of audiences, look for visuals that will not discredit your message. There is no formula to predict what constitutes a familiar setting for a specific audience. Therefore, test the draft of your material with focus groups or by individual interviews with a sample of the intended audience. "Tell me what you see in this picture. What's it all about?" (See Chapter 10, Learner Verification.)

d. Bridge language barriers

Use visuals to help communicate with non-English-speaking patients. Figures 7-7 and 7-8 appear side-by-side in a book of illustrations for non-English-speaking patients. The book uses pictures and multi-language questions and text for assessment/admissions history, hospital directions, and physical examinations/ medical procedures. Instructions and additional aids are given in the Guide for follow-up of the questions.

2. Visuals can reduce the amount to be read

Visuals are much more effective than hard-to-read text; they help clarify steps in procedures and they can show concepts that are hard to put into words such as growth and development of the body.

a. Convert hard-to-read text to visuals

Administrative information is hard to read. Usually the document is long, without breaks; typically it has small print. Readers lose their place partway

FIGURE 7-7

Figure displays and communicates information helpful in a medical history. (*Source:* Do You Understand? [1989]: Literacy Volunteers of America, 5795 Widewaters Parkway, Syracuse, NY 13214)

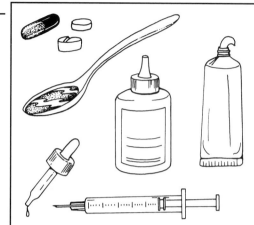

Suitable features for poor readers are:

- Clear line drawings of commonly used medicines
- Patient can point to the medicine being taken

FIGURE 7-8

Questions in six languages on medication patient is taking. (These accompany visuals in Fig. 7-7 above.) (*Source:* Do You Understand? [1989]: Literacy Volunteers of America, 5795 Widewaters Parkway, Syracuse, NY 13214)

Do you take medicine?

Cambodian

ខ្ញុំ ?

Laotian

ທານ ໄດ້ຫນ ຢາ ບໍ່ ?

Vietnamese

Ban có uống thuốc không?

Polish

Czy bierzesz lekarstwo?

(chĕ bēair·zhessh lech·carst·vaw?)

Russian

Вы принимаете лекарство ?

(vē pri·ni·má·yĕt·yĕ lyĕ·kărst·vŭ)

Spanish

¿Usted toma medicinas?

(ōō·stĕd tō·má mĕd·ē·sé·nŭs)

Suitable features for poor readers are:

- Corresponding text in six languages for help in asking questions through the document. Once this occurs, frustration sets in as the reader attempts to regroup and locate the correct line. The similarity of terms and the formal writing style make locating the reader's place in the text more difficult. Also, the subject matter and reading level are intimidating.

Examples of such documents include eligibility requirements for health services, advance directives in terminal illness, and participant responsibilities in WIC (Women, Infants, Children Program). However, the information has to be understood if people are to obtain needed services.

The following WIC list of *Home Delivery, Participant Responsibilities* is an administrative document typical of those used in the health care field. The original document in text form is shown first. This is followed by an alternative presentation of the same information in visual format with a minimum of text (Figure 7-9).

Home Delivery Participant Responsibilities (Original Text)

Listed below are responsibilities of a WIC participant in the home delivery system:

1. A participant must provide the local WIC clinic with good directions to the participant's home. A participant's home must have clearly marked house numbers.
2. A participant must have pets, such as dogs, tied up and away from the delivery person's path.
3. A participant may not ask the delivery person to deliver foods to a location other than the one on the DVR list.
4. A participant may not ask the delivery person to enter the participant's home.
5. A participant, parent/guardian, or alternate must be home the first delivery of each month to receive food.
6. A participant must show the ID/VOC card to the delivery person the first delivery of each month to receive food.
7. A participant may not ask the delivery person to sign the DVR.
8. A participant must be home or must make arrangements with an alternate to be at the participant's home for each delivery.
9. A participant must be courteous to the delivery person. A participant may not harm or threaten the delivery person in any way.
10. A participant must contact the local WIC clinic when any problems occur concerning the delivery person or with the foods delivered.
11. A participant may not ask the delivery person to exchange food or deliver items other than what is listed on the DVR.
12. A participant may not call the dairy or the state WIC office. A participant may call only the local WIC clinic with any questions or concerns.

Using a visual format, Figure 7-9 provides the same information as the list, but presents it in a more visible format and with a positive tone.

When it is not feasible to convert text to visuals, there is another step you can take. Examine the layout and see if you can make the page **look** easier to read.

Layout refers to the arrangement of the text and the visuals on the page—the way that they are laid out. For example, the text may be in columns, or the text may be placed around the page with a visual in the center, or the text may take up the entire page. If there is no relief from solid text, or if the page has an overload of text and visuals, the reader may be turned off by the "busy" appearance and may not bother to make the effort to read it. Layout can attract attention or turn readers off.

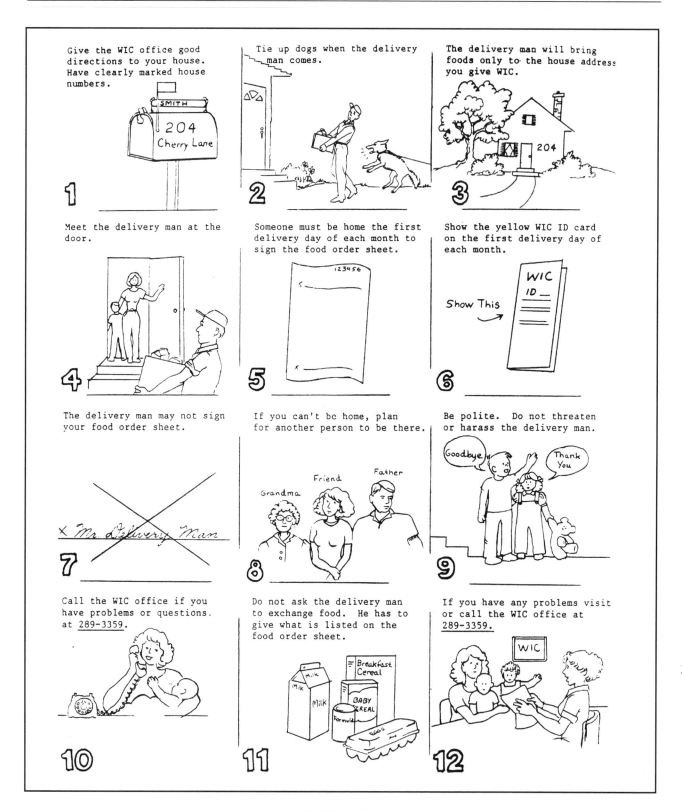

FIGURE 7-9

Responsibilities of a WIC participant in the home delivery system. Text and visual format. (*Source:* Visual format: Patricia J. Welch [1989]: L.D. GRADS Coordinator, Ashland Co. West Holmes Career Center, Ashland, OH 44805-9377)

What makes a page look easy to read?

IMPORTANT CHARACTERISTICS FOR LOW LITERACY PURPOSES:

- There is lots of white space to reduce distractions.
- The eyes travel easily across the page in a familiar pattern.
- Visuals have captions or cues to direct the eyes where to focus.
- Print size is at least 12 point, serif font.
- The page looks like it can be read in a few minutes.

b. Reduce text by illustrating the steps in a procedure

Procedural messages are the backbone of health care instructions. Visuals help reduce the reading to explain diagnostic tests, treatment procedures, and procedures for self-management. As shown in Figure 7-10, *place the visual adjacent to its corresponding text* when you are teaching a procedure so that the reader will make an immediate association. Figure 7-10 *shows* the person undergoing the procedure.

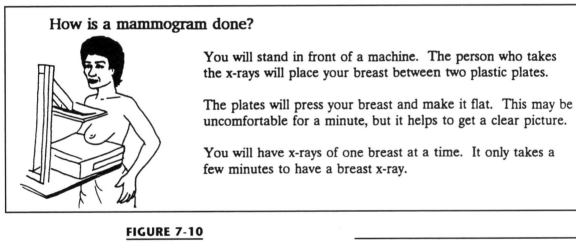

How is a mammogram done?

You will stand in front of a machine. The person who takes the x-rays will place your breast between two plastic plates.

The plates will press your breast and make it flat. This may be uncomfortable for a minute, but it helps to get a clear picture.

You will have x-rays of one breast at a time. It only takes a few minutes to have a breast x-ray.

FIGURE 7-10

An effective visual to explain a mammogram. Notice that the view of the woman facing the machine gives the full picture of what is taking place. (*Source:* West Virginia Cancer Information Service, Mary Babb Randolph Center, Morgantown, West Virginia 26506)

Suitable features for poor readers:

- Line drawing, no distractions.
- Illustration shows what the words describe.
- Visual helps patient to anticipate the experience.

FIGURE 7-9 (p. 102)

Suitable features for poor readers:

- The behavior in each item is visualized. If you can't read well, you still get the message.
- Each picture is numbered to help the reader keep her place on the page.
- The language is friendly and courteous; words are shorter.
- Less text to read; it also *appears* easier to read.

In the next example, Figure 7-11, notice how the *visuals work with the text* to help the reader understand the preparation for giving herself an insulin shot.

A note of caution: The authors have reviewed many instructions where the visuals are placed after the text or on separate pages, usually without captions or explanations. This creates problems: the readers may not know what parts of the text apply to what parts of the visuals, or they may skip the pages following the text. Sometimes the page with the visuals becomes separated and the patient doesn't see it at all.

Using visuals with other media: Combine a pamphlet and a demonstration with a poster or a flip chart to make procedures easier to understand. The pamphlet or instruction sheet provides the basic information. The demonstration shows how to apply it and provides the third dimension for size, shape, and "feel." The visual (poster or flip chart) helps reinforce and clarify the key points.

FIGURE 7-11

Part of a sequence of steps in an easy-to-read diabetes instruction. (*Source:* Understanding Diabetes Mellitus. Buffalo Veterans Administration Medical Center, Buffalo, NY)

Suitable features for poor readers:

• Drawings are next to the related text.
• Visuals emphasize key behaviors.
• Clear background keeps focus on key behaviors.
• Text sequence is numbered.
• Sequence is easy to follow.

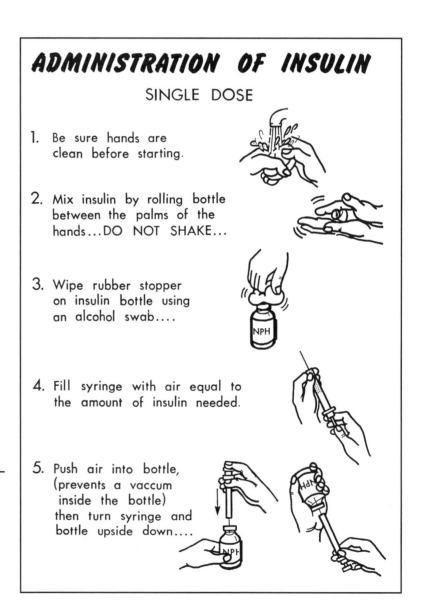

ADMINISTRATION OF INSULIN

SINGLE DOSE

1. Be sure hands are clean before starting.

2. Mix insulin by rolling bottle between the palms of the hands...DO NOT SHAKE...

3. Wipe rubber stopper on insulin bottle using an alcohol swab....

4. Fill syringe with air equal to the amount of insulin needed.

5. Push air into bottle, (prevents a vaccum inside the bottle) then turn syringe and bottle upside down....

c. Show contrasts in growth and development

Concepts of growth and development are hard to put into words. Visuals help people establish in their minds the location of an internal organ or body opening. Be sure to include enough of the outside of the body because that is the beginning point for easy identification. Cross-sectional views and anatomical drawings from medical textbooks are seldom suitable for patients with low literacy skills.

Figure 7-12 is a series of visuals to show contrasts that help patients understand the stages of growth and development of a fetus during pregnancy. Think of the number of words you'd have to use to show this!

Use visuals effectively: Internal parts of the body "come alive" when models made of synthetic material are used to explain a procedure. For example, if you are teaching a part of the body that is unfamiliar, such as the rectum, use a visual (chart or poster) first to orient the patient to the body. Then use a model as a detailed visual to provide the specific information and to stimulate questions from the patient.

Models give a three-dimensional perspective that helps in understanding size and shape. Some models, such as those for teaching breast self-examination, are also useful to teach patients the tactile sense.

FIGURE 7-12

An effective visual showing the growth of the fetus. (*Source:* Program for International Training in Health [INTRAH]. Teaching and Learning with Visual Aids. London, Macmillan, 1987)

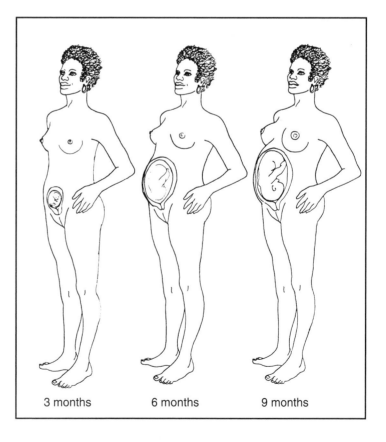

3 months   6 months   9 months

Suitable features for poor readers:

- Realistic line drawing of entire body makes it easier to perceive changes.
- Consistent position of mother promotes faster identification of fetus.
- Clear background, no distractions.
- Matches the logic and experience of the reader.

3. Provide visual cues and interaction

Visuals attract attention and help the reader focus on what is important. Four examples will help you select ways to give emphasis: use devices to call attention to key points; use action captions; introduce color; and provide the reader with a chance to interact with the instruction.

a. Use visual devices (cues) to call attention to key points

Call attention by directing the eye where to look in the visual. This step is a remedy for the random eye movement and the lack of attention to detail discussed earlier.

There are a number of devices you can use: arrows, underlining, circling, magnifying the text, boxes, a spash of color—they all help to cue the eye where to look.

Try asking the patient to do the underlining or circling with your guidance. If you are using only a small portion of a long instruction, consider cueing that portion so that the patient can quickly access the right part.

In Figure 7-13, which one of the ways to emphasize a key point will you use?

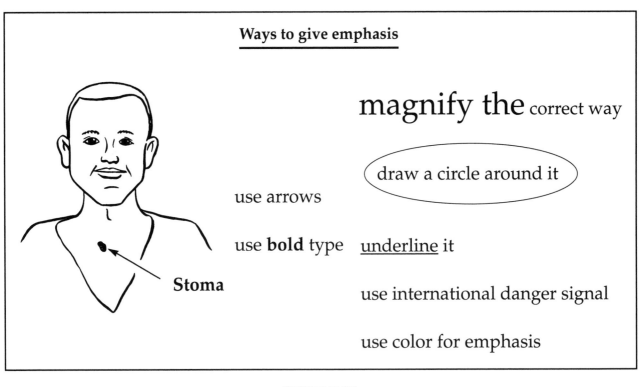

FIGURE 7-13

Devices to call attention to key points. Consider using one of these to help keep attention focused on your message.

b. Use action captions for emphasis

Because they are short and look easy to read, captions are often read before the text. Together with the visual, that may be all that a reader looks at on a page. So write captions that help people remember the key points. Captions are effective when they do one of the following:

- Tell what to look at in the visual
- Point out what is significant, new, different
- Point out what the implications are

In Figure 7-14 the message is *do not change the positioning of the seat belt after it is fastened.* The action captions beneath each of the four illustrations explain why it is important to keep the seat belt positioned properly. Ordinarily we suggest showing only the right way so as to avoid confusion. But when you are changing a familiar habit, such as the way you wear your seat belt, you need to help the reader remember why it is wrong to change the positioning of the belt. Readers will stay interested in captions for as long as three lines of about 15 words per line.[20]

FIGURE 7-14

Action captions as part of each picture. Arrows and magnification are used to draw attention to the snug fit of the seat belt. (*Source:* Consumer Information Department of Transportation, NHTSA, November 1992)

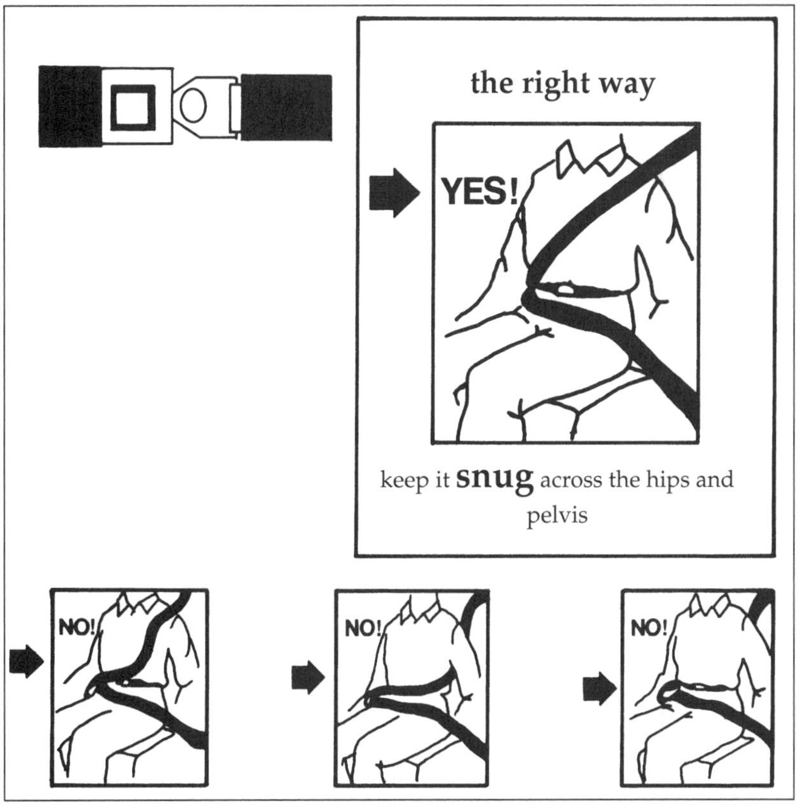

the right way

YES!

keep it **snug** across the hips and pelvis

NO! — Not across your stomach because you may get hurt here

NO! — Not under your arm because you can hurt your ribs and insides

NO! — Not behind your back because you will fall forward

Suitable features for poor readers:

- Text gives reinforcement.
- Arrows call attention to "Yes" and "No."
- For emphasis the right way is magnified.

c. Use color for emphasis

Color is compelling in its ability to attract and hold attention and is therefore a very appropriate way to give emphasis to key points.

Use color to highlight and for a number of other reasons, such as to differentiate, to add clarity, to help focus the eye, and to be realistic. For example, in a visual of a catheter kit, one color could be used to identify which parts must be kept sterile. When the instruction is in black and white and you wish to call attention to one key message, use a fluorescent marker. Keep color in balance with the whole instruction so that it does not become a distraction.

Age, gender, and ethnic preferences for color vary markedly. Test your choices of color with a sample of the intended audience. Pettersson brings out how people in different cultures and socioeconomic groups use colors in different ways and with different meanings.[21]

The colors at the center of the visible light spectrum—white, yellow, and green—are the most visible. Note that road signs are often black on yellow—the colors with the most visible contrast. The least visible colors are red, blue, and violet.

d. Use interaction to give emphasis to key points

Visuals that ask the reader to respond by doing something give emphasis by implanting the message in the memory. Several ways are listed below to illustrate how you can build interaction into your instruction by having the patient do something. Place a check mark by one or more that you think you might use:

___ Have patients place an "X" through pictures of high-fat foods to differentiate from low-fat foods.
___ Have patients check off on a diet list the foods they'll buy.
___ Have patients mark a calendar to keep track of pills or medication.
___ Show patients where to underline the key points in the pamphlet.
___ Show a picture that asks patients a direct question: "What/how/when are *you* going to do . . ."?

When you have decided what you are going to use for interaction, get feedback from the intended audience on their opinions of it. Use a focus group or individual interviews. Figure 7-15 was presented to a focus group for their reactions. It shows four different ways of reminding women to take their birth control pills. The first two examples use a didactic approach. The third example uses one interaction, while the fourth uses two interactions.

4. Use visuals to provide motivation

The following four ways of using visuals to provide motivation are especially useful for poor readers: use visuals for the cover; use visuals in a comic book style or a photo novella; use testamonials; try a visual or graphic type of game.

FIGURE 7-15

The focus group selected the fourth example as the most suitable (shows calendar and pill box with two interactions). (*Source:* Program for International Training in Health [INTRAH]. Teaching and Learning with Visual Aids. London, Macmillan, p. 119, 1987)

Special features for poor readers:

- Patient interacts by marking on calender pill taken each day (3).
- Patient marks calender as in (3) and also marks in pill box the pills taken each day (4).

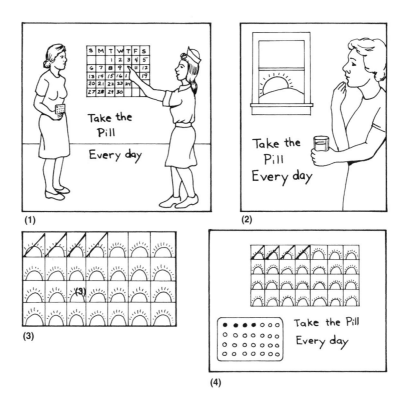

a. Use a visual on the cover to motivate the reader

The cover is the face of your material; it must be appealing while providing a good idea of the subject. Because reading is not easy for poor readers, they need more of a nudge to get them to open the page. The cover has to deliver that nudge.

The cover should tell the purpose at a glance, and it sets the tone and mood for the instruction. It needs to attract and hold attention long enough to get the reader into the material.

The style of artwork should lead to the readers' recognition and identification with the subject. Sketches of friendly people or realistic line drawings with blank backgrounds are easily recognized. Abstract or stylized graphics lack realism and are not likely to be seen as relevant by poor readers. Photographs are an attractive medium, but most of them include too much unneeded detail. Details tend to distract poor readers and they may never "see" your message. Simple line drawings work better. Keep them basic and uncluttered.

Figures 7-16, 7-17, and 7-18 are covers from three pamphlets, all dealing with the same subject of eating habits/weight loss. As you look at each one, consider the points made in this section about covers. Check which you think would be most suitable for poor readers. The authors' answers are provided.

Which Covers Are Most Suitable for Poor Readers?

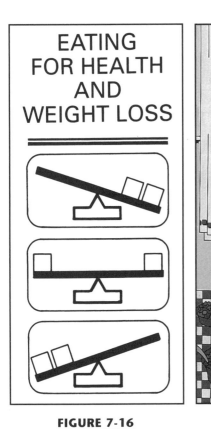

FIGURE 7-16

(*Source:* Bob Palaski Assoc., Silver Spring, MD)

Suitable

____ yes ____ no

FIGURE 7-17

(*Source:* National Cancer Institite, National Heart Lung & Blood Institute, NIH Pub. 88-3000)

Suitable

____ yes ____ no

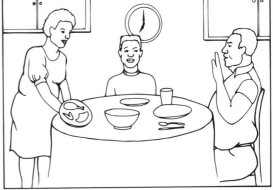

FIGURE 7-18

(*Source:* Health Literacy Project, Health Promotion Council of Southeastern Pennsylvania, Inc., Philadelphia, PA)

Suitable

____ yes ____ no

ANSWER TO COVER QUIZ

Fig. 7-16: No. Abstract symbols are hard to interpret.

Fig. 7-17: No. Unclear purpose and too many distractions.

Fig. 7-18: Yes. Communicates purpose immediately.

b. Use visuals to tell a story

Why are comic books so popular? They are visual! As brought out by Migdol (1961), comic books lend themselves naturally to five measures of effective communications: easy readability, flow, crispness, clarity, and color.[22]

There are two important reasons to use a picture/story for health education purposes: (1) people remember stories better than a set of facts; (2) using familiar characters in a familiar setting can help people talk about the real problems in their own lives and community. Following are some examples:

1. A local legend for Native Americans, "Old Man Coyote and Turtle Woman" is used in a modified comic book format about fetal alcohol syndrome for pregnant women.[23]
2. A series of comic booklets model the way a mother could talk to her son about AIDS.[24]
3. A modified comic book is the central feature of a series of learning aids to motivate pregnant teenagers to eat healthy foods.[25]
4. The photo novella concept (photographs used in a comic book format) is being used more widely for empowerment.[26] Although used widely with Hispanic populations, some Hispanic populations are not familiar with it. Test the concept before using it. Figure 7-19 attracts your attention with its scenes and leads the reader into the message quickly.

c. Use visuals for testamonials

Visuals give realism to testamonials. You actually see the people talking. And testamonials are an effective way to build self-efficacy. They build upon the inference, "If your friends and people like you can do it, you can do it too." Testamonials may have greater influence than previously realized. A survey of mothers in the WIC program revealed that they preferred and trusted other mothers as the most reliable source of nutrition and health information.[27]

Testamonials are effective for people of all ages. An illustrative example is shown in an educational student magazine and a videotape on drug abuse

FIGURE 7-19

Health tips for adolescence are interwoven in the story of two sisters. (*Source:* A Time for Change. National Cancer Institute, NIH Pub. 88-2466)

Suitable for poor readers for these reasons:

- Realism through visuals.
- Captures and holds attention.
- Health message is woven into relevant life situations.
- Easy-to-read language and short conversational sentences.

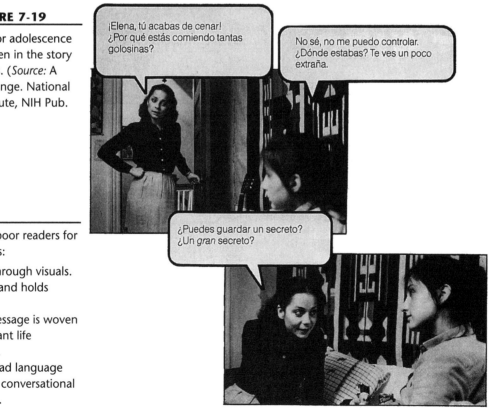

written and produced by sixty 8th graders (Figure 7-20). Furthermore, the testimonial format, multi-color, multi-sized print fits their culture and communication style. This student developed article, *If You Change Your Mind*, resonates like rock music.

c. Use graphics in a game format to motivate patients

Information learned in a game format that uses life experiences appears to be better remembered than traditional text. Graphics and visuals add realism to games that present concrete actions and relevant events. That is why they are likely to be remembered longer.[28] They also demand interaction and sharing in a social context. Games create a relaxed mood for learning.

Why do teenagers say yes?

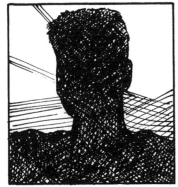

"Summer school of 6th grade I tried my first hit of marijuana someone turned me on to (it), a friend of mine did"

Teenagers have many reasons for saying "yes" to drugs. Saying yes can appeal to many things that people feel are important. "Just Saying 'No'" is not always so easy. It is helpful to understand the reasons why people say yes in order to have better reasons for saying no.

"I had a girl-friend that introduced me to cocaine and she said *'try this'* and I did."

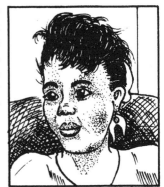

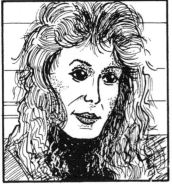

"A friend of mine would break into his dad's liquor cabinet and we'd drink beer together out in the cornfield."

"I started using drugs because of peer pressure, at the age of 13 years old."

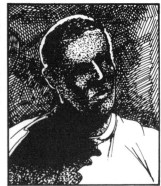

FIGURE 7-20

Effective drug abuse message for 8th graders. One of 16 pages that uses testamonials to appeal to teenagers not to use drugs. (*Source:* If You Change Your Mind. National Institute on Drug Abuse, NIH Pub. 93-3474, 1993)

Suitable for poor readers for these reasons:
- Faces give emphasis to message.
- High emotional impact.
- Creditability is apparent.
- Matches logic and experience of readers.

Figure 7-21 is designed for an exhibit at health fairs to stimulate interest among Alaska Natives in eating healthier foods to prevent cancer. When tested with young adults, the question-and-answer game format received their enthusiastic approval.

FIGURE 7-21

Handouts and tip sheets on nutrition are used with the game format. (*Source:* National Cancer Institute, Branch of Special Populations, 1993)

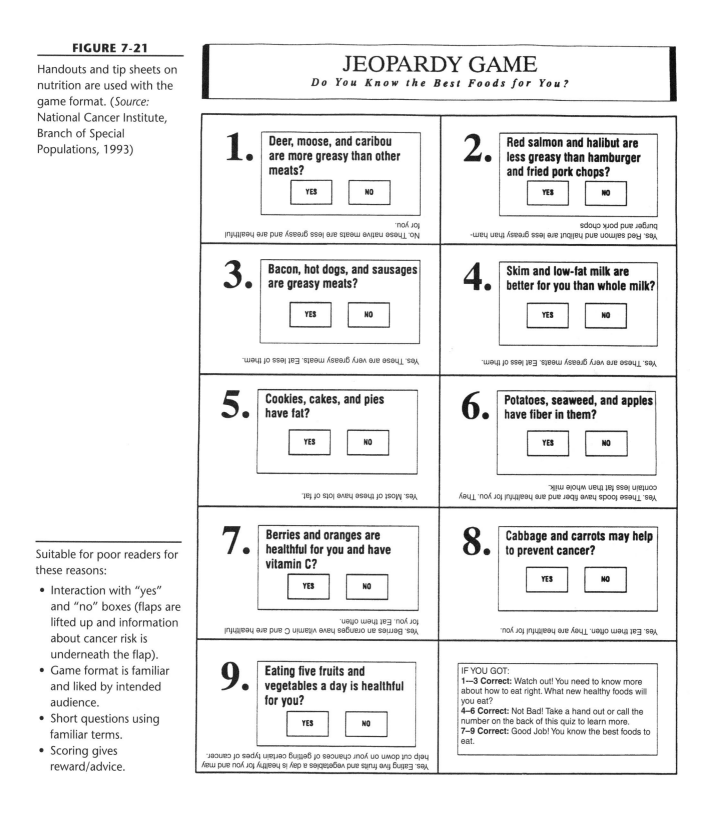

Suitable for poor readers for these reasons:

• Interaction with "yes" and "no" boxes (flaps are lifted up and information about cancer risk is underneath the flap).
• Game format is familiar and liked by intended audience.
• Short questions using familiar terms.
• Scoring gives reward/advice.

A note of caution: Select games that are popular with the intended audience and that require only one or two actions by the players. Combine other media such as handouts or pamphlets as take-home materials. Be sure to give explicit instructions on how to play the game. If scoring is a part of the game, keep it simple. Relate the interpretation of the score to the need for further information or advice. Test the concept and the draft of the game with the intended audience before using it. When games are used as exhibits they stimulate interest.

In conclusion, consider how you can achieve these outcomes:

___ Concentrate on main message.
___ Reduce the amount of reading in text.
___ Provide visual cues and interaction.
___ Provide motivation.

Part 3: Making Lists Understandable

Lists, graphs, and other stylized displays of information are widely used in the health field. Some are easy to understand and personalized; they build on patients' existing knowledge and use interaction. Other kinds of lists are hard to understand; they require the patient to match columns, integrate new information, and have complex displays, making it hard to access the information. Few lists contain directions on how to read them. Part 3 discusses both the easy- and the hard-to-understand lists.

Practical design and layout features can make access to information quick and satisfying to the patient. What are the more important design and layout features? The key design and layout features for easy understanding of lists are:

1. One central purpose
2. Directions on how to read them
3. Information limited to a specific objective
4. Easily recognized way to proceed in locating information
5. Patient interaction with the information presented
6. Familiar information that ties to existing knowledge

Four examples of how to make lists understandable

Each example illustrates four or more of the features listed above. Each example serves a different purpose, so the layout changes to suit the purpose of the list.

Example 1: The central purpose in this list, Figure 7-22, is to find out if you have gum disease. The directions tell you what to do and the language is easy to understand. It's short, and when you finish you know what to do. You also know what your risks are if you don't take action.

Example 2: Lists can help the person know what specific behaviors to change by reading them at a glance. Figure 7-23 and Figure 7-24 are diabetic

FIGURE 7-22

Interactive list—good example. Suitable for poor readers for these reasons:

• Directions clearly tell that **any** symptoms require action.

• Only six items are displayed,

• Patient interacts with information.

(*Source:* Keep Your Teeth for Life. Maine Department of Health Services, Division of Dental Health, Maine AHEC System, Augusta, ME 04333)

Do You Have Gum Disease?

Anyone can get gum disease and not know it.
Gum disease is often painless.

Check to see if you have any of these:

❏ 1. Red, puffy gums that bleed when you brush your teeth
❏ 2. Gums pulled away from your teeth.
❏ 3. Pus between your teeth and gums.
❏ 4. Bad breath.
❏ 5. Loose teeth.
❏ 6. A change in how your partial denture fits.

If you checked *any* of the boxes above, you may have gum disease.
See a dentist to find out. If it isn't treated, it often gets worse. Teeth

diet lists that provide immediate feedback to the patient based on that patient's diet history.[29] Called "Steps to Better Health," these figures use the outline of footprints for display of information.

As the dietitian takes the diet history from the patient, she writes the *most critical changes* that the patient needs to make inside the "Steps" outline. After counseling the patient is given the "Steps" to take home. Patients put the information on the refrigerator for daily reference. Experience with four years of using the "Steps" shows that the patients do use them. They return to the clinic with the "Steps" in hand for an update. It is a list that they have had a part in constructing.

Example 3: Lists are one of the early forms used in teaching people to read and write, so the concept of simple lists tends to be familiar to poor readers. The function of lists as we generally use them is to *do everything* on the list, such as shopping lists—"things to do." This same type of list works in health care instructions.

Figure 7-25 is an example of a list where the person follows the directions as given in the list. Information is limited to a few steps organized by when to do them. A key point is that the patient is told when to stop one procedure and begin a new one.

Example 4: The last example of lists suitable for poor readers are those that provide new information in the context of what people already know. This approach has two positive features:

1. It is quickly to understood because it contains familiar information.
2. It builds self-efficacy by acknowledging that people already know quite a bit.

FIGURE 7-23

Diet list blank form. Steps before the clinic visit. (*Source:* Janet Weiner, Metro Health, Maternity and Infant Care Program, 3104 W. 25th St., Cleveland, OH 44109)

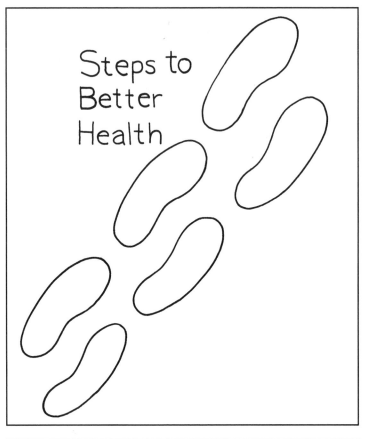

FIGURE 7-24

Diet list personalized with an example of the changes a patient needs to make. (*Source:* Janet Weiner, Metro Health, Maternity and Infant Care Program, 3104 W. 25th St., Cleveland, OH 44109)

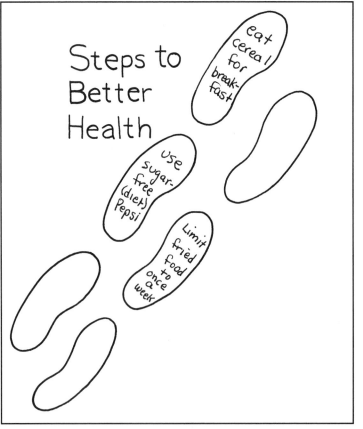

FIGURE 7-25

Effective instruction for treatment of sprain injury. Suitable for poor readers.

When you have an arm or ankle sprain, do this:

For the first 3 to 5 days

1. Keep the arm or ankle raised above the level of your heart.
2. Do not use the sprained ankle or arm:

   Ankle—use crutches, don't put your weight on it.
   Arm—use the sling and the splint at all times.

For the first day and a half: Apply ice to the sprain for 30 minutes every 2 hours.

After the day and a half: Stop the ice. Apply heat for 15 minutes four times a day.

After 5 days if you are still having discomfort, please call me at

_____. My name is

_____

Continued pain may mean you need further treatment and evaluation.

Do not use the injured arm or ankle as long as it is painful.

FIGURE 7-26

Effective list to create awareness of foods that have fat. It builds on what people already know. (*Source:* Why All the Talk About Fat? Native American Group. National Cancer Institute, Branch of Special Populations, 1992 draft)

Fat Foods

You probably know that these foods have a lot of fat:	You may not know that these foods have a lot of fat too:
• Butter	• Fry Bread
• Margarine	• Nuts
• Shortenings	• Chips
• Fat on meat	• Cheese
• Skin on Chicken	• Whole Milk
• Skin on Turkey	
	• Gravies
	• Sauces
• Lard	• Ice Cream
• Mayonnaise	• Cream
• Oil	• Donuts
• Salad Dressing	• Cakes
• Cookies	• Pies
	• Bologna
	• Hot Dogs
	• Hamburgers

Figure 7-26 is a simple *standardized* list intended to teach people to identify foods that are high in fat. Like the other examples, it has one central theme and has an easily recognized way to proceed in locating information. Although there are more than 10 items displayed, they are "chunked" into two main groups, one of which "you probably already know about" and one which "you may not know." Additionally, the foods are chunked according to the way that people think about them. Designed and tested with a Native American population, it was perceived by them to be "the best page" in a several-page booklet.

The four examples of lists suitable for poor readers have several points in common: they have a central purpose and an easily recognized way to proceed in locating information. They are easy to use and do not require extensive directions on how to access the information. They have been found useful by patients.

When do lists become hard to understand?

They become hard to understand when they display a volume of different kinds of information requiring the reader to perform a series of tasks to obtain the information. Usually they do not give explanations of where to start and how to proceed in reading the list. These lists reinforce "What's the use? I can't do it" attitudes.

What can you do if you have a complicated list? Try to simplify the list by breaking it into several bite-size pieces such as in the previous four examples. If that isn't feasible, then write step-by-step directions on how to use the instruction, where to start, and how to proceed. This is easier to say than it is to carry out because of our own familiarity with the subject and the detailed process being asked of the readers. The following information is intended to help you get started in writing directions.

How to write directions

First: "Walk through" all of the explanations and steps that need to be taken to understand and use the list. Unless the purpose is *explicitly* stated on or near the list, you may have to write in the purpose. The purpose should be stated in terms of the *patients' use* or the problem that the list can help the patients solve.

Next: Write the first step. Tell where the patients enter the list. Do the patients always enter it at that point? Or is it only an intermediate step?

Then: Proceed to explain each following step in a similar manner. If appropriate, include an example.

Finally: Explain what the patients end up with, and how they use that information.

For lists that are very simple, short, with one central function of six or less items, some of the above steps may be dispensed with. But think back to the last time you assembled some simple purchase that came unassembled in a box with assembly instructions. The author of that instruction thought it was simple!

Figure 7-27 is an example of a hard-to-understand diet list from a currently used patient instruction about sodium. No directions were included with the diet list. Figure 7-28 shows directions developed by the authors to explain how to use the diet list.

Testing directions: One way to test your directions for completeness and suitability is to ask a few patients to carry them out *exactly* as you have written them. Make notes of where they begin to hesitate and become confused. These are places that need revision or examples.

FIGURE 7-27

Diet list on sodium content of foods. Example from a currently used patient instruction about sodium. Patients need help understanding how to use the numbers to make correct food choices, and they need examples of what meals for one day might be like.

Sodium Content of Common Foods Diet List

How much is *too much*?
- A safe amount of sodium is 1,100–3,000 milligrams (mg) a day.
- The average American consumes 2,000–7,000 mg of sodium per day!
- Just one teaspoon of salt contains over 2,000 mg of sodium.

Sodium Content of Common Foods (mg)

MILK GROUP	MG SODIUM	PROTEIN GROUP	MG SODIUM
Ice cream, 1/2 cup	50	Dried beans/Peas cooked, 1 cup	5
Milk (whole, low-fat, skim)	125	Meat, fish, poultry (plain), 2 oz	50
Low-fat yogurt, 8 oz	175	Processed cheese, 1 oz	400
Natural cheese, 1 oz.	175	Peanut butter, 4 Tbsp	320
Eggs, 2 large	120	Instant pudding, 1/2 cup	470
Cottage cheese, 1/2 cup	460	Dried beans/peas canned, 1 cup	850
Luncheon meat, 2 oz	450	Hotdog, 2	1,257

GRAIN GROUP		FRUIT AND VEGETABLE GROUP	
Pasta, rice, cereal, 1/2 cup (cooked without salt)	5	Fresh, canned, or frozen Fruits & juice, 1/2 cup	2
Bread, 1 slice	120	Fresh, frozen vegetables (plain) 1/2 cup	5
English muffin	150	Canned vegetables, 1/2 cup	200
Cereal (dry) 3/4 cup	200	Tomato or vegetable juice 1/2 cup	400
		Sauerkraut, 1/2 cup	750
		Pickle, 1 large	1,400

OTHER FOOD GROUP			
Gingerale, 12 oz	20	Cookies, 2	100
Tonic water, 12 oz	20	Salad dressing, 1 Tbsp.	150
Cola (regular)	25	Catsup, 1 Tbsp	156
Cola (diet), 12 oz	30	Apple pie (1/8)	200
Butter, 1 tsp	40	Corn chips, 1 oz	230
Margarine, 1 tsp	50	Danish, 1	250
Bouillon cube	420	Bacon, 2 slices	275
Soup (canned) 1 cup	1,000	Soy sauce 1 tsp	343
		Baking soda, 1 tsp	821

FIGURE 7-28

Directions for understanding how to use the sodium list, Figure 7-27. (*Source:* C. Doak, L. Doak, J. Root)

DIRECTIONS: How to use this list to keep your sodium down

Purpose of the list: You need to cut down on sodium. Consider cutting down to a teaspoon of salt, a goal of 2,000 mg a day. An easy way to do this is to eat foods low in sodium.and go easy on foods high in sodium. This list will help you do that by telling you how much sodium you are getting when you eat certain foods. Try to skip foods with the large sodium amounts—the large numbers. Big numbers are bad for you.

What is on the list: It shows the names of meats, fruits and vegetables, breads, milk, and other foods that you eat a lot. After each food is a number that tells you how much sodium is in one serving of that food. The measurements for the amount of foods may be different. Sometimes the serving is for a cup (c), a tablespoon (Tbsp), a teaspoon (tsp), or an ounce (oz).

Where should I begin? Start up at the top on the left where it says Milk Group. Read through the whole page, all the lists. Then think about which of these foods you eat a lot. Each food has a different amount of sodium. That's the number to the right of the food.

Then what do I do? Go back to the Milk Group heading.

Step 1. Go through the whole list again, but this time *put a line under the foods you want to eat* for breakfast, lunch, supper, or snacks.

Step 2. Now look at the numbers on the right side of each of these foods you underlined. *Make a list of these numbers.*

Step 3. *Add the numbers on your list.* If your total is more than 2,000, you'd get too much sodium. If your total is less than 2,000, you are doing okay. Go back to the list and change some of your foods so that you end up with a total of 2,000 or less for everything you eat or drink each day.

More about what makes lists hard to understand: Figure 7-27 requires the person to concentrate on just one subject, the sodium content of foods. Lists that require the person to concentrate on as many subjects simultaneously have a task demand far beyond the skills of poor readers. Even the skills of many good readers can be taxed.

For illustrative purposes the authors present two lists containing information that require the reader to perform similar complex tasks. The first one, reading a bus schedule (Figure 7-29), is a test question from the National Literacy Survey. This is considered a difficult question; it is at level 4 on a scale of 1 to 5 (see Chapter 1). Only 18 percent of adult Americans could do this task correctly.

VISTA GRANDE

This bus line operates Monday through Saturday providing "local" service
to most neighborhoods in the northeast section
Buses run thirty minutes apart during the morning and afternoon rush hours Monday through Friday
Buses run one hour apart at all other times of day and Saturday
No Sunday, holiday or night service.

OUTBOUND
from Terminal

INBOUND
toward Terminal

You can transfer from this bus
to another headed anywhere
else in the city bus system

Leave Downtown Terminal	Leave Hancock and Buena Ventura	Leave Citadel	Leave Rustic Hills	Leave North Carefree and Oro Blanco	Arrive Flintridge and Academy	Leave Flintridge and Academy	Leave North Carefree and Oro Blanco	Leave Rustic Hills	Leave Citadel	Leave Hancock and Buena Ventura	Arrive Downtown Terminal
AM											
						6:15	6:27	6:42	6:47	6:57	7:15
						6:45	**6:57**	**7:12**	**7:17**	**7:27**	**7:45** Monday through Friday only
6:20	6:35	6:45	6:50	7:03	7:15	7:15	7:27	7:42	7:47	7:57	8:15
6:50	**7:05**	**7:15**	**7:20**	**7:33**	**7:45**	**7:45**	**7:57**	**8:12**	**8:17**	**8:27**	**8:45** Monday through Friday only
7:20	7:35	7:45	7:50	8:03	8:15	8:15	8:27	8:42	8:47	8:57	9:15
7:50	**8:05**	**8:15**	**8:20**	**8:33**	**8:45**	**8:45**	**8:57**	**9:12**	**9:17**	**9:27**	**9:45** Monday through Friday only
8:20	8:35	8:45	8:50	9:03	9:15	9:15	9:27	9:42	9:47	9:57	10:15
8:50	**9:05**	**9:15**	**9:20**	**9:33**	**9:45**	**9:45**	**9:57**	**10:12**	**10:17**	**10:27**	**10:45** Monday through Friday only
9:20	9:35	9:45	9:50	10:03	10:15	10:15	10:27	10:42	10:47	10:57	11:15
10:20	10:35	10:45	10:50	11:03	11:15	11:15	11:27	11:42	11:47	11:57	12:15
11:20	11:35	11:45	11:50	12:03	12:15	12:15	12:27	12:42 p.m.	12:47 p.m.	12:57 p.m.	1:15 p.m.
PM											
12:20	12:35	12:45	12:50	1:03	1:15	1:15	1:27	1:42	1:47	1:57	2:15
1:20	1:35	1:45	1:50	2:03	2:15	2:15	2:27	2:42	2:47	2:57	3:15
2:20	2:35	2:45	2:50	3:03	3:15	3:15	3:27	3:42	3:47	3:57	4:15
2:50	**3:05**	**3:15**	**3:20**	**3:33**	**3:45**	**3:45**	**3:57**	**4:12**	**4:17**	**4:27**	**4:45** Monday through Friday only
3:20	3:35	3:45	3:50	4:03	4:15	4:15	4:27	4:42	4:47	4:57	5:15
3:50	**4:05**	**4:15**	**4:20**	**4:33**	**4:45**	**4:45**	**4:57**	**5:12**	**5:17**	**5:27**	**5:45** Monday through Friday only
4:20	4:35	4:45	4:50	5:03	5:15	5:15	5:27	5:42	5:47	5:57	6:15
4:50	**5:05**	**5:15**	**5:20**	**5:33**	**5:45**	**5:45**	**5:57**	**6:12**	**6:17**	**6:27**	**6:45** Monday through Friday only
5:20	5:35	5:45	5:50	6:03	6:15						
5:50	**6:05**	**6:15**	**6:20**	**6:33**	**6:45**						Monday through Friday only
6:20	6:35	6:45	6:50	7:03	7:15						

To be sure of a smooth transfer
tell the driver of this bus the name
of the second bus you need!

On Saturday afternoon, if you miss the 2:35 bus leaving
Hancock and Buena Ventura going to Flintridge and Academy,
how long will you have to wait for the next bus?

A Until 2:57 p.m.

B Until 3:05 p.m.

C Until 3:35 p.m.

D Until 3:57 p.m.

E I don't know.

FIGURE 7-29

Test question used on National Literacy Survey. (*Source:* Adult Literacy in America, National
Center for Literacy Statistics, U.S. Department of Education, 1993)

The second illustration is a diabetic diet list intended for low literacy patients. Like the bus schedule, it displays a large volume of imformation requiring matching and acculmulating facts. The patient is asked to use the booklet to select foods for three meals and three snacks each day. Figure 7-30 is one page of: "Lunch" from *Eating Healthy Foods* prepared specifically for those clients who have minimal reading skills.

Each list was evaluated using four variables related to the difficulty of using the lists:[30]

1. Multiple feature matching
2. Complex displays involving information nested within the display
3. Number of distractors
4. Conditional information that must be taken into account in order to arrive at a correct response

A comparison of the variables for the two graphics is shown in Table 7-2.

The reader must integrate information and draw a number of inferences to reach a decision in using the bus schedule as well as the diet list. These are skills that four out of five Americans have not mastered. Health instructions that use such a highly complex format make learning *how to learn* as difficult as having the medical problem.

Sometimes designers of health instructions assume that pictures in color overcome the complexity of the format and the volume of information. This

TABLE 7-2

Comparison of complexity of bus schedule with diet list

VARIABLES ASSESSED	BUS SCHEDULE	DIET LIST
1. Multiple-feature matching	Saturday afternoon Leaving Hancock and Buena Ventura Arriving at Flintridge and Academy Calculate wait time	Match food symbols on plate with food symbols on list Locate amount recommended for each serving of each food group Select number of foods from each food group on list Match with diet prescription Check with other meals for accuracy
2. Complex displays involving nested information	Columns of departure and arrival locations and of times	Columns of foods with 5–6 pictures per column Amounts change with each picture Modifers for foods (raw, cooked)
3. Number of distractors	Other destinations and terminals	Plate with food, utensils, placemat Color code (six colors) Food symbols
4. Conditional information to be taken into account for correct response	Information at top of page, in fine print, contains the critical Sat. schedule modifier	Exchange one food for another within same food group using correct serving amount for each food Cook foods using patient's correct fat allowance

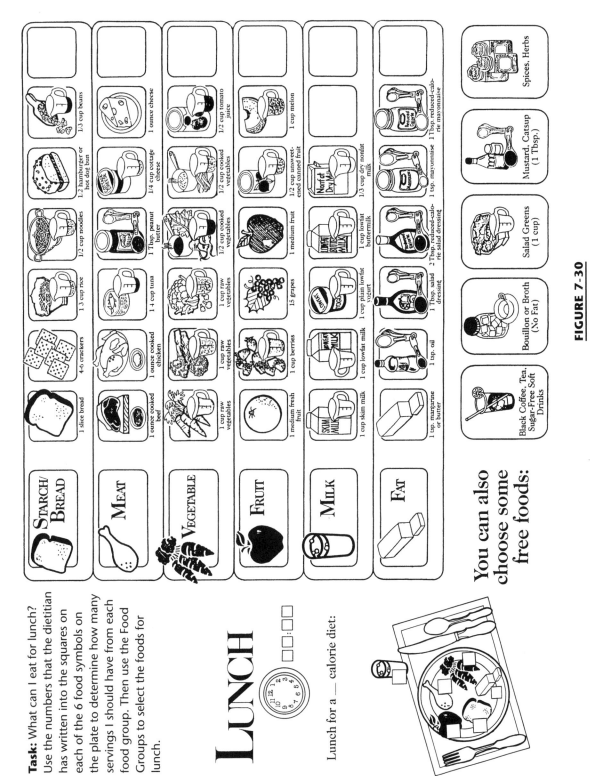

Task: What can I eat for lunch? Use the numbers that the dietitian has written into the squares on each of the 6 food symbols on the plate to determine how many servings I should have from each food group. Then use the Food Groups to select the foods for lunch.

LUNCH

Lunch for a ___ calorie diet:

STARCH/BREAD

1 slice bread | 4-6 crackers | 1/3 cup rice | 1/2 cup noodles | 1/2 hamburger or hot dog bun | 1/3 cup beans

MEAT

1 ounce cooked beef | 1 ounce cooked chicken | 1/4 cup tuna | 1 Tbsp. peanut butter | 1/4 cup cottage cheese | 1 ounce cheese

VEGETABLE

1 cup raw vegetables | 1 cup raw vegetables | 1 cup raw vegetables | 1/2 cup cooked vegetables | 1/2 cup cooked vegetables | 1/2 cup tomato juice

FRUIT

1 medium fresh fruit | 1 cup berries | 15 grapes | 1/2 cup cooked fruit | 1/2 cup unsweet-ened canned fruit | 1 cup melon

MILK

1 cup skim milk | 1 cup lowfat milk | 1 cup plain lowfat yogurt | 1 cup lowfat buttermilk | 1/3 cup dry nonfat milk | 1/3 cup dry nonfat milk

FAT

1 tsp. margarine or butter | 1 tsp. oil | 1 Tbsp. salad dressing | 2 Tbsp. reduced-calo-rie salad dressing | 1 tsp. mayonnaise | 1 Tbsp. reduced-calo-rie mayonnaise

You can also choose some free foods:

Black Coffee, Tea, Sugar-Free Soft Drinks | Bouillon or Broth (No Fat) | Salad Greens (1 cup) | Mustard, Catsup (1 Tbsp.) | Spices, Herbs

FIGURE 7-30

Diet list for low literacy patients. (*Source:* Eating Healthy Foods: A Guide to Good Eating [1988]: American Diabetes Association Inc. American Dietetic Association, Alexandria, VA.)

is a false assumption. Pictures in color attract attention, but the reader still has to have the skills to work with the variables assessed in Table 7-2.

What are more effective ways of teaching a number of complex concepts? Several chapters in the book deal with this subject as well as Part 2 of this chapter. One solution is to partition the information into several smaller and simpler displays as the *unit* of information. It is important to use a format that the patient is familiar with so that he doesn't have to learn the format as well as the information it contains with the variables assessed in Table 7-2.

For example, Figure 7-31 is one sheet in a series that the diabetic patient can use for planning his meals. The intent is to communicate the information

FIGURE 7-31

One-day meal plan for a diabetic Hispanic client. Suitable for low literacy patients. (*Source:* California Diabetes Program, CA Department of Health, Sacramento, CA)

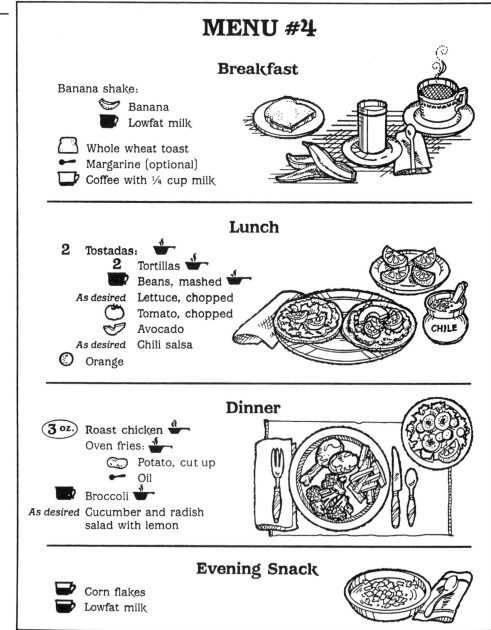

in units of *one day at a time.* Included with the series is a *key sheet* that explains the symbols and how to use the sheets.

"How-to-use-it" directions are almost always needed regardless of the format of the list or chart. Poor readers need to have each step explained. Figure 7-28 is a good illustration of the amount of detail needed in the directions.

Graphs are another source of problems for poor readers

Graphs are often used to plot weight gain in pregnancy as well as for other purposes. Because graphs are abstract, require matching different kinds of information, and are not perceived as real, they do not communicate well to poor readers. Figure 7-32 compares the patient's weight gain over time with the ideal weight gain. First the patient determines her current weight gain by subtracting her previous weight from her current weight. Originally, the next

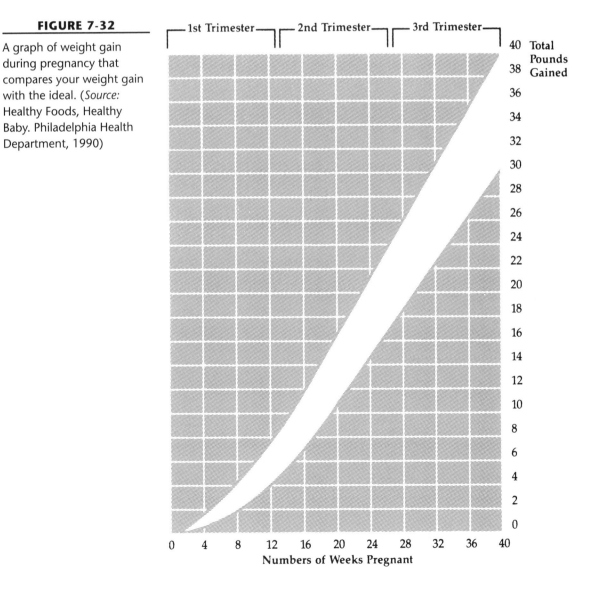

FIGURE 7-32

A graph of weight gain during pregnancy that compares your weight gain with the ideal. (*Source:* Healthy Foods, Healthy Baby. Philadelphia Health Department, 1990)

step called for the patient to plot her weight gain on the graph. This step turned out to be too difficult for pregnant teenagers even after the graph and the steps were explained.

Two changes were made: the nurse or nutritionist now records the patient's weight gain on the graph instead of the patient; and the graph itself was changed to show a wide line through it representing the right range of weight gain. Staff have found the graph useful in counseling to dramatize the weight gain for patients who need special attention.[31]

The problem is that many people, especially poor readers, do not understand the *logic* of this type of format. Interpreting a comparison from a graph requires *skills of inference* that many poor readers have not developed.

A simple list in which the patient records her monthly weight gain is suggested instead of a graph. On the page opposite the graph (Figure 7-32) contained in the booklet *Healthy Foods, Healthy Baby* a simple record of the patient's weight goal, the current date of weight, the patient's weight, and the number of weeks pregnant can be recorded by the patient (Figure 7-33 below). Experience in using this type of list shows that it is a more suitable format than having patients attempt to use the graph itself.

Summary

As a concept, lists have advantages over long paragraphs of text. Lists are pre-organized, which helps to reduce the sheer volume of information. They help with quick recognition of the information should the reader skim or later

_____

FIGURE 7-33
_____

A simple way for the patient to record and keep track of her weight gain during pregnancy. A poster of this graphic could be placed above the scale in the clinic. (*Source:* Healthy Foods, Healthy Baby. Philadelphia Health Department 1990)

My weight gain goal is _____ pounds.

Date	My Weight	Weeks Pregnant
_____	_____	_____
_____	_____	_____
_____	_____	_____
_____	_____	_____
_____	_____	_____
_____	_____	_____
_____	_____	_____
_____	_____	_____
_____	_____	_____
_____	_____	_____
_____	_____	_____
_____	_____	_____
_____	_____	_____

review the material. Many complex lists used in health care instructions are not understood, and to make matters worse, they do not contain "how to" instructions or examples. Gillespie (1993) helps professionals understand graphics with a succinct review of research.[32]

To make lists suitable for low literacy patients:

___ State the purpose explicitly.
___ Limit information to a specific objective.
___ Write detailed directions for patients' use.
___ Encourage patient interaction, or give an example of how to use the list.
___ Provide an easy way to proceed in locating information.
___ Verify your directions with a few patients.

Take your pencil and check the features you want to include in your next design of lists.

References

1. Visuals as used in this chapter refer to pictorial images. Graphics refer to stylized designs and layout (lists, charts).
2. Vogel DR, Dickson GW, Lehman, JA (August 1986): Driving the audience action response. Computer Graphics World. As contained in Pettersson R (1989): Visuals for Information: Research and Practice. Englewood Cliffs, NJ 07632: Educational Technology Publications, p. 73.
3. Wileman RE (1993): Visual Communicating. Englewoods Cliffs, NJ 07632: Educational Technology Publications.
4. White JV (1988): Graphic Design for the Electronic Age. New York: Watson-Guptill, 211p.
5. Petterson R (1989): Visuals for Information: Research and Practice. Englewood Cliffs, NJ: Educational Technology Publications. See Chapter 2: Perception, learning and memory, p. 73.
6. McBean G, Kaggwa N, Bugembe J (1980): Illustrations for Development. Nairobi: Afrolit Society. WASH Tech. Report 24, USAID, Department of State.
7. Pretesting and Revising Instruction of Materials for Water Supply and Sanitation Program, WASH Tech. Report 24, October 1984, Office of Health, Bureau for Science and Technology, USAID, Task B-339, Camp Dresser & McKee, Inc., 1611 North Kent St., Room 1002, Arlington, VA 22209.
8. Werner D, Bower B (1982): Helping Health Workers Learn. The Hesperian Foundation, PO Box 1692, Palo Alto, CA 94302.
9. Teaching and Learning with Visual Aids. INTRAH. Program for International Training in Health, Katherine Murphy (ed). Materials Unit, INTRAH, School of Medicine, University of North Carolina, Chapel Hill, NC (1987).
10. Audio Visual Communications Handbook, Dennis W. Pett (ed). World Neighbors, International Headquarters, 5116 North Portland Ave., Oklahoma City, OK 73112 (1976).
11. Beyond the Brochure: Alternative Approaches to Effective Health Communication (1994): Centers for Disease Control and Prevention, Atlanta, and AMC Cancer Research Center, Denver.
12. Jonassen DH (1982): The Technology of Text: Principles for Structuring, Designing, and Displaying Text. See Chapter 5, Brain functions during learning: implications for text design, pp. 91–120. Englewood Cliffs, NJ 07632: Educational Technology Publications.
13. Ibid., p. 99.
14. Schramm W, Roberts D (eds) (1971): The Process and Effects of Mass Communication. Urbana, IL: University of Illinois Press. As quoted in Hicks RC: (1977): A Survey of Mass Communication, p. 306. Gretna, LA: Pelican Publishing.

15. Mackworth NS, Bruner JS (1970): How adults and children search and recognize pictures. Human Development 13:149–158. As quoted in Vernon MD (1973): Visual Perception and Its Relation to Reading, p. 5. Newark, DE: International Reading Association.

16. Ley P, et al. (1976): A method for decreasing patients' medication errors. Psychological Medicine 6:599–601.

17. Ley P (1977): Psychological studies in doctor patient communication, pp. 19–29. In Stanley Rachman (ed), Contributions to Medical Psychology, vol. 1. Oxford: Pergamon.

18. Rogers E, Shoemaker F (1971): Communication of Innovations, 2nd ed. New York: Free Press. See Chapter 3, The innovation decision process.

19. Bandura A, (1977): How individuals, environments, and health behavior interact: social learning theory. As contained in (1990): Health Behavior and Health Education: Theory, Research and Practice, Glanz K, Lewis FM, Rimer BK (eds). San Francisco: Jossey-Bass.

20. White JV, Ref. 4, pp. 124–126.

21. Petterson R, Ref. 5, Chapter 4, Designing visuals for information, pp. 250–253

22. Migdol MJ (1961): Comics as a public relations tool in communications. Master's thesis, University of Buffalo, Buffalo, NY.

23. Old Man Coyote and Turtle Woman. Community Health, Crow Indian Hospital, Crow Agency, MT 59022.

24. Mom and Son. Native American Women's Health Education Resource Center, PO Box 572, Lake Andes, SD 57356-0572.

25. Healthy Foods, Healthy Baby. Maternal and Infant Health, Department of Public Health, Philadelphia, PA 19146.

26. Wang C, Burris MA (Summer 1994): Empowerment through photo novella: portrait of participation. Health Education Quarterly 21(2):171–186.

27. Nitzke S: Reaching low literacy adults wiith printed nutritional materials. Journal of American Dietetic Association 87(9): Supplement: S73-S77.

28. Coleman JS (August 1973): The Hopkins Games Program: conclusions from seven years of research. Educational Review, pp. 3–7.

29. Weiner J, Senior Nutritionist, Metro Health Maternity and Infant Care Program, 3104 West 25th St., Cleveland, OH 44109.

30. Adult Literacy in America, National Center for Education Statistics (1993): GPO Stock 065-000-00588-3, Section III-91.

31. Scharf, M (1994): Division of Maternal and Child Health, Philadelphia, PA 19146. Personal communication.

32. Gillespie C (1993): Reading graphic displays: What teachers should know. Journal of Reading, 36(5): 350–354.

8

"What kinds of instructions work best—pamphlets, audio tapes, or video?"

Teaching with Technology

This chapter is intended to excite you and involve you in the use of technology in your patient education endeavors. You are already familiar with and probably use at least some of the technologies described in the following pages. We explain the technology, its applications, and details for your use in teaching your patients.

We begin with one of the simplest teaching technologies—audiotaped instructions (Part 1)—and proceed to the use of television (Part 2), and finally to interactive multimedia (Part 3). These technologies, especially multimedia, are moving forward at a rapid pace and are increasingly used in education. They can multiply your teaching effectiveness and increase your patients' ability to learn.

Part 1: Audiotaped Instructions

Listening, rather than reading, is a more natural way to understand language. Kavanagh writes that, "Listening is easy; reading is hard."[1] Patients have told us, "I pay attention more and don't get lost when I hear it on the tape." In addition to the information content, word-sounds convey emotion and cultural messages that affect our willingness to learn and believe.

One-to-one oral instruction is the most common communication medium in health care, but it takes time—an increasingly scarce commodity at busy clinics. And when oral instructions are given, the research shows that patients forget most of what they have been told within minutes after leaving the clinic or doctor's office.[2] Audiotaped health care instructions may overcome these problems and they offer additional advantages.

129

Although audiotaped health instructions are becoming more common, especially for health promotion and disease prevention, many health care providers are not yet using them to teach patients. However, the authors have found that with as little as an hour of training in the development and use of audiotaped instructions, providers can produce highly effective instructions and they develop great enthusiasm for the medium. By participating in the exercises presented in the pages that follow, you will learn quickly and have a similar enthusiasm for audiotaped instructions—and so will your patients.

The rationale for this part of the chapter is to provide you with both the learning principles and the detailed "how to" guidance to enable you to make your own tapes and use them to teach patients. Objectives for Part 1 are:

- To apply the education principles discussed in Chapter 2 to making your own audiotaped instructions
- To provide details on how to make your own audiotaped instructions and use them to teach patients effectively
- To provide an understanding of audiotape and tape players

The imperative for audio

For the approximately 27 million adults in the United States who are functionally illiterate, audiotaped instructions may be one of the few ways that health care messages can be understood.[3] They rarely choose print formats as a source of information; even simply written instructions may be discarded. In addition to the 27 million are another 45 million adults with marginal literacy skills.

Audiotaped instructions can reach these populations. For example, during 1990 and 1991 the public health nurses in Trinidad–Tobago found that their printed leaflets were not influencing many parents to bring their preschool children in to be immunized against measles. Many of the parents, especially those living in the hills, could not read the leaflets. So, the nurses used a school choir to make an audiotape of the immunization messages. The 30-second song was played often over local radio stations. Nearly everyone has a transistor radio, and the messages got through. Soon, children everywhere were singing a new song, "Zap! Goes the Measles" (to the tune of "Pop Goes the Weasel") and immunizations soared. Their song:

> *For if you were like nature boy*
> *You'd never get the measles.*
> *But if you are more normal-like*
> *Here comes the measles.*
> *To keep you from all harmful things*
> *You see it is so easy;*
> *So we will do what doctor says . . .*
> *"Immunize" (doctor's voice)*
> *Zap! Goes the measles!*

In the above example, the children's voices were instantly recognized and accepted by their radio listeners. Acceptability of your health care messages can be enhanced by having them recorded by those of your target culture.

A growing number of audiotaped health care messages are now in use in the United States. Many are innovative and use talk-show formats or rap songs to convey health care or prevention messages about breast self-examination, smoking cessation, and healthy weight loss.[4,5,6] See Figure 8-1.

Learning principles for audiotaped instructions

The learning theory and principles described in Chapter 2 apply to audiotapes as well as other methods of communication. To learn to apply them, the authors ask you to engage in brief exercises as we proceed. By the end of the chapter you will understand the principles for teaching with audiotapes, and will have attained skills to develop your own instructions in this medium.

Limit the objectives

This rule is especially critical for audiotapes because the attention span for listening is so limited. Tapes of one to five minutes hold attention and are more effective than longer tapes. King (1979) and others have found that even with the added stimulus of visuals (educational television), a break is needed every eight minutes if learner attention is to be maintained.[7]

FIGURE 8-1

Smoking cessation package: audiotape and pamphlets. (*Source:* Basel Pharmaceutical and American Lung Association)

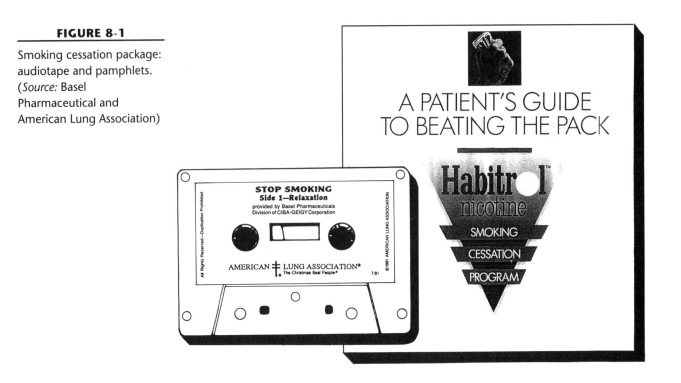

For short taped messages, one objective is preferable (two at the most). A single objective has the virtue of leading to a smaller number of details in the content of the audiotape, which reduces the chance for information overload. Thus, the message has a better chance of being remembered.

Many currently available audiotaped instructions in the health field have too many objectives and hence are too long. The "rule of seven" (see Chapter 5) is violated and the listener soon realizes that there is no way to follow along.[8] It's a little like trying to drink out of a fire hose—a gulp or two may be possible, but there is no way to keep up! Besides, long tapes are nearly always dull tapes.

EXERCISE ON LIMITING OBJECTIVES

Select an over-the-counter or a prescription medication and read the label and patient package insert (PPI). (Note: If you prefer, in lieu of medication label and PPI, for this series of exercises, you can use an instruction you are developing or using with your patients.) List the possible objectives for a short audiotaped instruction for patients. You may include such objectives as how to take the medication, possible side effects, what to do if . . . , and purpose of the medication—all worthy objectives.

Next, select one or two of these objectives that are most critical in terms of patient knowledge and behavior. These objectives will be the basis for an audiotape. How will you deal with any topics you have left out? If necessary, include them in a short supplemental handout, or make a second tape.

Focus on behaviors

Since so few points can be presented during a short audiotape, focus on the key behaviors rather than facts. Increase motivation by presenting information in the sequence of the Health Belief Model[9] (see Chapter 2).

EXERCISE ON BEHAVIORS

Make a list of the patient behaviors needed to meet the objective(s) you identified in the previous exercise. Now arrange these behavior topics in a Health Belief Model sequence (see Chapter 2 for sequence). Select only enough topics to make a tape of about three minutes.

Make it interactive

As noted in Chapter 3, interaction is a key instructional component to achieve comprehension and recall. Consider building interaction into audiotaped instructions by using (1) a dialogue format, (2) a question-answer (Q/A) format, (3) a supplemental medium such as a booklet or picture sheet to be marked in response to questions or cues on the tape.

Dialogue commands listener attention even on subjects about which listeners have little interest. Many aspects of the "overheard conversation" are inherent in dialogue and these tend to capture listeners' attention.[10] Unless there is a compelling reason not to use dialogue, it should be the first choice for tape format.

The Q/A format offers a structure to present new information and to obtain interaction and feedback. The Q/A responses may be generated by two voices on the tape: perhaps the health care provider and a client. A more direct interaction with the listener may be obtained by posing questions directly to the listener, pausing, and allowing time for the listener to respond verbally. For example:

"We've talked about several foods you should not eat. Now which of those foods will you cut from your meals?" (5–10-second pause). "If you said . . . , you are right!"

Supplemental materials such as true/false, fill in the blanks, circle the right picture, or other paper and pencil responses can provide the interaction that leads to learning. Such supplemental materials may be locally produced and consist of a single sheet of paper.

Existing pamphlets or booklets may also be used, with the client given instructions on the tape as to the page and action required. A pause must be built into the tape to allow time for the client to respond. An audiotape would be an excellent medium to "walk" a newly diagnosed diabetic patient through with directions on how to use a chart or a food exchange list.

EXERCISE TO MAKE INSTRUCTION INTERACTIVE

Continuing with the earlier exercise, develop listener interaction on the key points you've already listed. Use (1) a direct question(s) to ask on the tape; (2) ask the listener to respond to the questions in a supplementary material that is used with the audiotape.

Key points first and/or last

Stating the key point(s) last is more important than stating them first for audiotaped messages. The listener may not be paying attention at the start and may have missed the key message. But a compelling dialogue may have captured attention during the running of the tape, and the ending message will be heard.

Unlike the printed page, which can be referred to over and over again, audio instructions played over radio stations must usually be grasped at once unless the message is given a rerun. Thus, by repeating the key point(s) of your message first and last, you will better assure that listeners get the message.

EXERCISE ON WRITING THE OPENING AND CLOSING STATEMENTS

Write a short statement in narrative style that gets right to the point or purpose. This will be the opening and closing statement on your audiotape. The message need not be worded exactly the same in both places, but the idea should be the same. For example, an opening message: "I hear I can get AIDS by sharing needles. Is that true?" An ending message: "Clean your needles with bleach. It can save your life."

If you have performed each of the four exercises above, you now should have the draft of an effective health care instruction for the medication (or other topic) you have selected. You are now ready to record the message.

Recording the message

Since high fidelity is not needed for speech, you can use an inexpensive portable cassette recorder/player. Set the volume control near the high end, and hold the microphone about 16 to 24 inches (40 to 60 cm.) from the speakers' faces. Press the record control(s) and talk naturally. Be careful not to speed up your rate of speaking. After you have recorded the message, rewind and replay your message to assess how it communicates.

The dialogue should come in short, natural chunks; there should not be long paragraphs of spoken information without intervening responses. As in ordinary conversation, the responses may be very brief and consist of no more than "Oh?" or "H-mm!" "Oh, I see," or "How?" If you are not satisfied with some part of the recording, record it anew—it takes only a few minutes. A summary of the process to plan and make audiotapes is shown in Box 8-1.

In ordinary conversation we often speak in incomplete sentences; we interrupt, we respond to show we understand (or don't), and we may repeat a part of what the first speaker has just said. In your recordings, give free rein to these natural characteristics of speech. If necessary, some of these can be edited out later.

BOX 8-1

Procedure to make an audio taped instruction

1. Select a health care area or disease category as a subject. Topics such as nutrition for diabetics, smoking cessation, or hypertension are suitable.

2. Decide on an objective(s) that could be covered in this short tape.

3. List the topics that must be covered to meet the stated objective(s), and arrange the topics in accordance with the sequence suggested by the Health Belief Model.

4. Decide on the key message for the beginning and the ending. Write statements for the topics. You may prepare a written script or only list the topics and talk extemporaneously. A rough outline of the topics to be covered in the dialogue and who is to speak is sufficient. The topics may be arranged in a time-line diagram as shown in Table 8-1.

5. Begin recording using your script. If speaking extemporaneously, start by reading the opening statement, and then proceed as you would in talking about each topic with a friend or a client.

6. Play back the tape. Revise if needed. Test it with a few patients.

During our workshops, the above process is completed by small groups in less than an hour. Participants are under time pressure to do so. The time pressure creates some anxiety, and speaking into a microphone adds anxiety for many as well. Since time permits only a rough outline, nearly all recordings are extemporaneous. You may be encouraged to know that although many enter into this exercise with some anxiety and reluctance, all are enthusiastic about the results they have achieved when they hear their recording aired immediately afterward over the PA system.

Script vs. extemporaneous recordings

Although there is much more vitality and humanness in extemporaneous recordings, many prefer to read from a script. The dilemma here is that although scripts make the recording more predictable, most scripts sound like a written speech that is read. The language tends to be more formal, it lacks interest, and the literacy demand is higher. A nurse who faced this dilemma found a reasonable solution that may be helpful:

"I just can't write a script that sounds natural. All my education has taught me to write in a formal style. But I found a way to overcome it. When I'm going to talk to a new patient, I often make a list of the subjects I want to cover. When I see the patient, I take a tape recorder along with me and turn it on. I soon forget the recorder. After the session is over I transcribe and edit the tape to take out the 'errs' and 'ahhs' and I've almost got a finished script."

Another way to obtain a natural-sounding script is to use a small focus group from the intended audience to read your draft script aloud. Then ask, "How would you say that if you were talking to a friend?" Proceed to revise the script using the audience's words in place of yours, except where they would be wrong.

Extemporaneous expressions and recordings can have an excitement that captures and holds the listeners' attention. Listeners overlook minor imperfections and indeed see them as human qualities. Sometimes, even on their first try, recordings by health professionals achieve drama and high believability.

Converting a pamphlet to an audiotaped instruction

You can use an existing pamphlet or other written instruction as a starting point to produce an outline or script for an audiotape. This is especially easy to do when the pamphlet presents information in a question-answer format, or already contains dialogue.

When using a pamphlet as a starting point, one must guard against trying to include on the tape all the factual information shown in the pamphlet. Stay with the central objective; omit all or nearly all other information.

Comprehension of audio instructions

Factors that *favor* comprehension and acceptance of audiotaped instructions:

1. Listeners respond to the dynamics of the spoken language.
2. People with low literacy skills can understand words and concepts at higher rates for speech than they can read in text.
3. Decoding of spoken words may be simpler than decoding for reading.
4. Common words are used more often in speech than in text.
5. Speech—especially extemporaneously—carries more redundancy than text.

Let us examine each of these in turn. First, the **dynamics of spoken language.** All of the emotional and dramatic characteristics of speech are available on audiotaped instructions. The voice may be soft and confident to inspire trust, or imperative to inspire the need to act. Speech rate can be varied to give emphasis to the more important facts. These qualities are difficult or impossible to achieve with text.

Platt[11] (1992) describes how the voice can convey empathy, which is especially important when the client or patient is angry and needs to be reassured that you understand. Such reassurance can deflect a patient's anger so that any subsequent verbal transaction becomes more rational and productive.

Svarstad and Mechanic[12] (1976) point out motivational benefits of speech when the physician speaks in an authoritative manner. In their study, such speech led to a 40-percent higher compliance among patients to take their medications as directed.

Earlier we mentioned the advantages of a dialogue format. Advertisers have used this dynamic for years. Consider the following typical television dialogue to sell laundry detergent—hardly a topic of high audience interest. The television scene is often set in a lady's laundry room, where her friend has just stopped by on her way home from shopping.

After stuffing several dirty shirts in her machine, the first lady reaches for a box of laundry detergent, but is stopped by the visiting friend who says, "Martha! You're not going to use that weak detergent on those dirty collars, are you!"

"Well, this is the kind of soap my mother always used."

"That won't do. Here! (reaching into shopping bag for a box of the sponsor's product). Try this. _____ will make those shirts whiter than white!" etc.

The advertisers know that the dialogue will keep the viewers' attention focused on the TV screen to listen in to this conversation. It is compelling. We too can use this format to gain and hold the attention of our patients.

Now, consider the **higher rates for speech.** Stitch and colleagues (1974) have shown that adults who have lower literacy skills, and who have no intellectual or hearing impairment, can understand spoken instructions at a much higher rate than they can read the same instructions.[13] This is a significant finding for health educators because:

- Verbal instructions can be presented at a normal speaking rate and still be understood by those with low literacy skills. Indeed, the message is best understood if presented at a normal speaking rate.
- If spoken instructions are said slowly, the listener will tend to focus on one word at a time, with the result that the listener forgets the words that were said earlier. Thus, although the listener hears and understands every word, the meaning of the sentences and the message is lost.

Decoding of spoken words is often less demanding for listeners. Words tend to be heard whole. Even when the listener is uncertain about the meaning of a word, the surrounding content and the syntax may help to convey or reinforce the meaning.

Common words are more frequently used in speech, especially informal speech. This effect can be seen by examining text where both narrative and nonnarrative paragraphs are used. The narrative, which uses active voice, almost invariably has many more common words.

Another way of examining this effect is to apply readability formulas to both kinds of text on the same subject, or even in the same document. The narratives, even those with longer sentences, have readability levels lower than the nonnarrative text. This point is illustrated by comparing text samples from a publication that includes both narrative and nonnarrative forms. The average readability level of a DHEW (Department of Health, Education, and Welfare) publication on alcohol and women is at the 12th grade. But the narrative parts, as shown below, are at about 6th-grade level.

"Work was good—it gave me a feeling of being alive. But when I would come back to my apartment, it was lonely and silent and dark. Finally, I got fed up and didn't go home after work at all—I'd go to a bar and stay 'til it closed."

—Toni, a high school teacher

Redundancy is usually considered a fault in documents though it is prevalent in speech. Redundancy makes understanding easier in spoken communications because it offers alternative opportunities and cues to understanding a message. Notice the redundancy and extra bridging words in this audiotaped conversation, where HCP is the health care practitioner and C is the client:

"CLEAN YOUR NEEDLES WITH BLEACH"

HCP:	First of all, don't share needles. But if you're gonna share, clean your needles with bleach.
C:	Cleaning . . . cleaning my needles with bleach?
HCP:	Yeah, clean your needles with bleach! Take your works—after you fix—pull bleach into the syringe, squirt it out. . . .
C:	What do you mean bleach?
HCP:	Bleach, regular household bleach, the kind you buy at the store.
C:	You mean like Chlorox?
HCP:	Yeah, Chlorox. . . .

Teaching with audiotapes

Teaching with audiotapes has much in common with other methods of instruction. As with other methods, taped instructions are most effective when preceded by a short preamble to provide the context for the message. This should state the purpose of the tape and the benefits to the patient. For example, a preamble for a tape about mixing baby formula might say:

"This tape will tell you how to mix the baby formula so it's just right for your baby. Please listen to the tape; then we'll show you how to mix the formula. The tape only lasts five minutes."

Teaching strategies will vary depending on where the taped instruction is being given and the form of any supplemental instruction. At outpatient clinics, patients can listen to the taped message over a special telephone as illustrated in Figure 8-2. The clinic receptionist invites each arriving patient to listen to today's health message and points to the telephone. "Just pick up the phone and listen," patients are advised. The tape-to-telephone system is low in cost and easy to install. It is described in more detail later in the chapter.

For in-patients, leave a portable tape player and earphones with the patient. Give the patient a brief introduction about the tape and show how to start, stop, and replay the message. A supplemental page may be given to the patient, perhaps with visuals, and blank spaces where the patient may write questions for later discussion with the nurse, physician, or nutritionist. Explain that the tape may be listened to as many times as the patient chooses.

An alternative is to play the tape over the audio channel that is a part of the TV/radio system at many hospitals. This approach eliminates handling the tape player with patients, but does require them to tune in at the scheduled times of play.

A taped instruction can be given to patients for home use. Many patients have tape players at home. An advantage of the take-home tape is that other

FIGURE 8-2

Tape-to-telephone use in a clinic waiting room

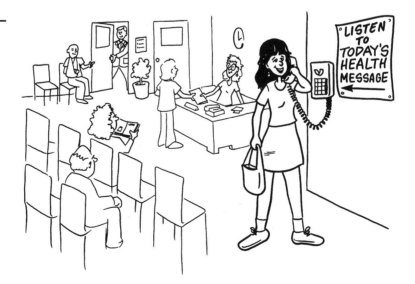

members of the patient's family may also hear it and thereby provide support. Audiotape cassettes cost less than a dollar (US), which is comparable to the cost of many pamphlets, especially pamphlets printed in color.

Making your own audiotaped instructions

A little planning makes the work go much easier. Consider enlisting the aid of others to plan and to make the tape with you. A colleague or a small committee can help by reacting to and offering fresh ideas. A committee is also a convenient source of voices for recording a dialogue.

As noted earlier, a productive way to begin is to write your objective (what you want the listener to do); then list the key points that will inform and motivate—better yet *involve*—the listener to take the desired actions. For example, for an audiotape on taking medication to reduce high blood pressure, the hypertensive patient might need the following:

- Motivation to cooperate with the treatment (motivating factors: personal risk and personal benefits)
- Instructions on how to carry out the behavior(s) required
- Information to understand the need for continuity of the treatment

Unlike text, audiotapes operate within some specific time limitation. Listeners tend to lose interest after five minutes, so each tape or tape segment should not exceed this duration. A time-line diagram can be helpful to visualize the time sequence of information (see Table 8-1).

TABLE 8-1

Time-line diagram for a one-minute tape on hypertension medication

SUBJECT/	TIME (SEC.)	TOPIC
Motivation	0	You have high blood pressure, and it could cause a heart attack.
		But if you take your pills *every day,* your risk of heart attack will be much lower.
Behaviors	10	Take one of these _____ pills three times a day. Take one pill before each meal with a little water.
		If you forget a pill, take it as soon as you remember it. But don't take more than three pills during any one day.
		You must keep on taking your pills even when you feel okay.
		Get a refill on your pills before your bottle is empty.
Understanding treatment and medication	35	You must take these pills every day for the rest of your life.
		Your blood pressure now is 170 over 95. This is too high. The pills will make it lower.
		Call the clinic or your doctor if you feel dizzy—like you might fall down. This sometimes happens. If it does, we may change the strength of your medicine.
		Don't take a risk! Take your pills every day.
End	60	The little booklet on **high blood pressure medicine** will tell you more about your medicine and possible side effects. Please turn to page 4 in this booklet. Read each question, and mark your answers on the page.

The monologue above could be easily converted to a more interesting dialogue format between a health care provider (HCP) and a patient (P). The reader is invited to convert the content above into a dialogue—perhaps to a question-and-answer format that can include some of the usual speech responses, like "uh-huh" or "okay." It might start with the patient asking:

P: Is it true that high blood pressure could cause me to have a heart attack or a stroke?
HCP: Yes, you're at risk for both.
P: Well, is there anything I can do about it?
HCP: Yes, etc. . . .

An audiotape can be especially effective when presented as an introduction or precursor to an educational intervention, for example, a teaching session between a nutritionist and a patient, or a group of patients. Patients may be asked to listen to the audiotape first, and perhaps make notes of questions they may have for the nutritionist. For example, a tape about getting people to change their eating habits to more nearly follow the recent national nutrition guidelines might be planned like this:

OBJECTIVE

To convince the target population to move toward the two key goals of the national nutrition guidelines:[14] eat less fat and eat more fiber.

KEY POINTS

- Cut the fat off meat before cooking.
- Cook with less fat; how to do it.
- Key foods to eat instead of other foods.
- Eat more foods that have fiber, such as . . .
- These can cut your risk of getting cancer.

INTERACTION

- Ask questions, via dialogue, on cutting fat.
- Ask about meals patients would prepare to obtain more fiber.
- Ask which high-fat food patients will eat less of.
- Ask listeners to make notes of questions they would like to ask the nutritionist.

Audiotapes and equipment

This section describes audiotapes and the recorder-player equipment. Fortunately, the tapes and the equipment are reliable, inexpensive, and quite simple to use. We recommend portable tape recorders–players such as those shown in Figure 8-3. The equipment shown is priced lower than US$50.

Several makes are available for each of the recorder-players in the figure. The larger equipment at the left, with the piano key tab controls, is easier to use, and tends to be more reliable than the smaller units. Controls usually consist of: Record, Play, Rewind, Fast Forward, Stop/Eject, and Pause. Some recorders offer the option of Voice Activation, which means that the player will start to record when sound is present, and will stop shortly after the sound stops. This feature may be convenient, but is not required.

Electrical power sources are from internal batteries, or from an external power adapter (usually included) that plugs into a standard AC wall socket. Thus, there is great flexibility for use for playback to patients at bedside or in the examining room using batteries, or, at a fixed office or waiting room site, operating on AC power.

Patients can *operate the tape player* directly to listen to the health message, or the tape player may be connected to a dedicated wall telephone in the clinic waiting room where patients can pick up the phone to listen. The receptionist may suggest to patients that they pick up the phone. Also, a sign may be placed above the phone—"today's message for your good health"—or a notice about a more specific health topic. Tapes may also be played over a public address system, or over the radio.

Nearly all recorder-players include a built-in microphone that may be used to record voice messages, sound effects, and music. To record a message, push the "Record" tab(s); place the recorder-player about 16 inches (40 cm.) away and speak in a voice that is meant to be heard. It is useful to record a few short test messages first and play these back at different volume control settings to find the level suitable for your voice.

Two tape speed settings, 1.2 and 2.4 inches per second, are options on some recorder-players. Either speed is suitable for voice recordings, but the 2.4 setting is better for music. At the slower speed (1.2), the tape time duration is doubled.

Digital tape-to-telephone systems

In recent years, highly reliable digital technology has come to the tape-to-telephone players. Here is how it works: A standard audio cassette tape with your recorded health message is plugged into a small digital box where it is auto-

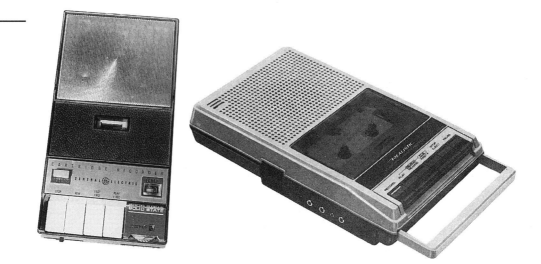

FIGURE 8-3

Inexpensive, portable recorder-players

matically stored in digital form. From that point on, when patients pick up the telephone to listen, the message comes from the digital memory and always starts at the beginning. There is no tape to rewind. You can set the telephone sound volume to whatever level is needed to be heard clearly, even in a noisy waiting room.

A digital tape player is shown in Figure 8-4. It is priced at about US$800. The equipment is about the size of a book and can be kept in a locked desk drawer. Your taped message can be changed in a minute by plugging in a new cassette.

Practical rules in selecting audiotapes

Select an audiotape size to fit your recorder-player. Standard-size cassette tapes are used in most medium- and larger-size portable players. These tapes are labeled C-30, C-60, or C-90 and indicate a combined playing time of 30, 60, and 90 minutes respectively for both sides (15, 30, and 45 minutes on a side). Since audiotaped instructions should be generally limited to about 5 minutes, the C-30 tapes provide ample run time.

Continuous-loop tapes do not require rewinding after each play, but play over and over again. This is a great advantage for settings where the tape player is to operate unattended, such as in a clinic waiting room. Tape durations of 30 seconds to up to 5 minutes are available.

Except for the continuous-loop tape, every tape has a short blank leader at the start. Nothing can be recorded on the leader. The leader is usually clear, as contrasted with the dark brown color of the active part of the tape, and typically has a 7-second run duration. When you plug in a new tape you must let the tape run until the leader has gone by before beginning your recording.

Digital equipment plays back a recorded message that has been stored in digital memory. As such, it does not use cassette tapes at all except as a means to insert the message the first time.

Audio cassettes, such as those shown in Figure 8-5, can be made tamperproof by breaking out the knock-out tabs using a small screwdriver or pocket knife. If you wish to later revise the tape, this can be done by first covering the knock-out tab holes using a small piece of cellophane tape.

FIGURE 8-4

Digital autoload tape-to-telephone equipment. (*Source:* Mackenzie Labs. Inc., Arcadia, CA)

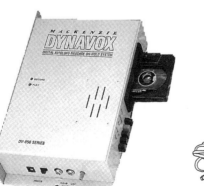
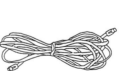
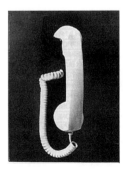

Should a portion of the tape become pulled out of the cassette, it can be rewound by inserting a finger or pencil eraser into one of the sprocket holes on the cassette and rewinding the loose tape.

Summary

Audiotaped health care instructions offer an effective approach to reach the 27 million functionally illiterate American adults. Tapes are also effective with the even larger number of marginally literate adults. The audiotape medium offers many advantages including the potential for cultural compatibility with target audiences.

Few commercially available audiotaped health instructions are suitable for patients with low literacy skills—indeed for any patients. You can easily plan and record your own taped instructions for use with your patients.

The educational principles described in Chapter 2 apply to taped instructions. A summary of these principles is:

- Limit objectives to what the client needs to know and do.
- Consider a sequence in accordance with the Health Belief Model.
- Include interaction with the listener.
- Tell the key points first and last.
- Consider using a dialogue format.

As teaching devices, audiotapes can be used alone or together with other modalities such as a related booklet or interaction sheet. Also, the tape may serve as a short introduction or refresher course prior to the patient seeing the nurse. The equipment to record and play audiotapes is inexpensive and is not difficult to operate.

Part 2: Teaching with Video

Television! Surveys tell us that most people spend several hours every day watching TV. May we assume that surely low literacy adults have no problem accepting and learning from this medium? As with other media, that depends on the video content and how it is used. We address selecting videotapes and methods to teach with television and interactive television so that patients accept and learn from it.[15]

FIGURE 8-5

Making tape cassettes tamperproof

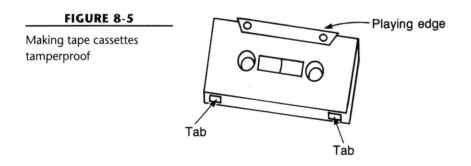

Playing edge

Tab

Tab

Video instructions for patients: What is available?

Impressive numbers of health education videos are available on a variety of subjects. Private sources and government agencies add to this number every week. A 1991 National Cancer Institute (NCI) directory offers over 100 patient education videos on cancer alone, and new videos are being produced for low literacy clients and various ethnic groups.[16] The NCI directory also includes a list of 37 vendor sources for patient education videotapes.

The purchase price for health care videotapes ranges from about US$20 to $350, with the average price a little under $100. Some sources also offer monthly rentals that are about one-quarter of the purchase price.[17] Many videotapes are available on loan from government and nongovernment voluntary agencies at no cost.

Local sources may offer budget-priced videos that are often highly relevant to local patient populations and ethnic groups. Production costs of some locally produced videos are quite low ($800–$3,000) and have correspondingly low purchase prices. Examples of these are: (1) "Put Away the Frying Pan," a low-cholesterol education video produced locally using a patient as the star, and (2) "Singing Eyes," a diabetes video narration that shows a series of culturally relevant (Navajo) images from 35mm slides.[18, 19] *A word of caution about "homemade" videos:* By now we are all sophisticated TV viewers and have high standards in terms of production quality. We are not turned off by simple videotapes that are well made, but an amateur video is no longer acceptable.

Selecting videotapes

Television is widely seen as an entertainment medium—we enjoy the story, the color, the action, the emotion, and the sound. Besides, we just watch and listen—we don't have to think or respond. Something more is needed when we want the patient to learn from the video. To select videos that patients are going to learn from, let us examine the characteristics that can make this happen.

Viewing time

Viewers at all literacy levels tend to lose interest in a video instruction after about 8 minutes.[20] Those with low literacy skills tend to lose interest even faster. Thus, videos with run times of 8 minutes or less are preferable. To maintain interest in a video with a longer run time, stop the video before 8 minutes and discuss the information presented thus far, or have the viewers fill in a few questions on a worksheet. Then resume the presentation.

When the video contains some humor and a number of scene changes that build interest, the viewers' attention can be held for more than 8 minutes. For example, a 13-minute video on mammograms involving a tense discussion, argument, humor, and scene changes can seem to have a shorter viewing time and thereby hold attention longer.[21]

Some videos can maintain interest for long periods by presenting an absorbing story line. The 30-minute video "Se Met Ko" presents an emotional human story about AIDS among a minority population in a large city.[22] The sequence of information follows the Health Belief Model (see Chapter 2): the risk of AIDS, how to prevent it, the prevention practices that are doable by the viewers, and the peace of mind when prevention actions are taken (the benefit).

Behavior focus

Select videos that focus on behavior changes and how to make these changes. Videos with a heavy factual content are boring to most people, and further- more, the viewer is soon overwhelmed with the sheer number of facts pre- sented and attention is lost. (See Chapter 5 for the limits on remembering items and facts.)

The authors have analyzed more than 50 health care videos. Some of them present over 60 facts in less than 15 minutes—a daunting memory task for any- body. Since the narrator rarely tells us which among the many facts are the most important, viewers try to remember everything—a frustrating experience.

Interaction

Select videos that offer some interaction with the viewer, either directly from the screen or indirectly by means of a worksheet. Interaction is important because it promotes attention and long-term learning. For videos that are suit- able except that they lack interaction, you can add some by making a short interactive worksheet that the patient responds to during or after the video showing. The worksheet should deal with a few key points or behaviors shown in the video.

Since low literacy patients tend to have a short attention span, the first interaction should occur early during the video run time—at the 4- to 6- minute point is about right. Subsequent interactions at 5- to 5-minute inter- vals should be planned. Some advertised "interactive instructional videos" run for 20 minutes or more before an interaction of any kind takes place. By that time most viewers' minds are elsewhere.

Other factors in the selection process

The images and people shown should be functionally and culturally appro- priate for your patient population. Examples of functionally inappropriate images: (1) a video on nutrition that shows many of the wrong food choices with equal emphasis on the right food choices, (2) a video to promote infant immunizations that portrays germs in the form of huge other-world monsters that few mothers would believe could possibly inhabit their infants.

Check the time allowed to read any text shown on the screen. Viewing time for text is often cut short—a problem for all viewers but especially for low literacy patients. If the viewing time is not sufficient for you to read with ease with time to spare, your patients won't be able to read the material and understand it.

When people from the target population are involved in writing the script, few if any uncommon words will be used. But when the script is entirely written by health professionals, "hard" words tend to creep in. The video announcers read these with great fluency and speed and the patients may be left behind. The unfamiliar medical words are not the only vocabulary problem. For example, a video on healthy teeth uses phrases and uncommon words in an unfamiliar context: "periodontal disease," "mainly related to," "frequency," "prone to."

Look for videos that employ dialogue rather than monologue speakers or presenters. Dialogue holds attention via the power of the overheard conversation. Monologue video instructions are inherently dull.

Pacing—the tempo and speed at which information is given—can be an important factor in the suitability of a videotape for patient learning. For a young audience, a lively pace and jazzy music may be more appropriate. This pace may be less appropriate for older audiences because they may not be as quick to pick up on the new information presented.

Additional methods to select videotapes

An approach to assessing suitability of a video is to use the 22-factor SAM instrument described in Chapter 4, or the checklist given at the beginning of that chapter. If you plan extensive use of a new video, field test the video with a small sample of your patient population as described in Chapter 10, Learner Verification. A more informal method is offered by Goldman and Zasloff (1994) based on a three-step active watching process.[23] The three steps are:

1. Describe what you see: say out loud or jot down what the video shows.
2. Identify the issues: the main point or theme, as well as more subtle issues such as feelings or cultural images.
3. After viewing, translate the message: in your own words. What does the message mean or tell you to do?

Based on what you've said or jotted down, and your translation, decide whether the video presents what you want to communicate to your patient population.

The Teaching Process

In what ways do you have to teach differently when low literacy patients are to learn from a video instruction? You might ask, "Teaching! But doesn't the video do the teaching? After all, that's its whole purpose." Unfortunately, a great many videos for patients don't deliver the teaching one hopes for and they are poorly suited for low literacy patients. These patients are not lacking in intelligence; they lack literacy skills and the experience that comes with those skills. To make video an effective teaching medium, consider the steps in Box 8-2.

BOX 8-2

Using video with low literacy clients

PREPARATION

1. Preview the video yourself and make a list of the key behaviors presented. Note any cues that point to these key behaviors so you can share these with your patients later.

2. Make copies of any lists or texts shown on the video for the patients as a paper copy handout.

3. Consider making a one- or two-page worksheet to obtain interaction with your patients during and/or after showing the video.

THE TEACHING/LEARNING SESSION

1. Preview the video for the patients. Tell them the purpose of the video in terms of its benefits to them. Tell them the main points/topics they will see, and how the video relates to other teaching materials such as pamphlets, booklets, lists, etc.

2. Explain the meaning of any uncommon words. (Use examples.)

3. If the run time exceeds 8 minutes, consider stopping the video and obtaining interaction with patients via discussion or a worksheet.

4. After the viewing, explain again the purpose and how the video can help them. Initiate a discussion about the video; its key points; how the viewers could (or could not) do what the video asks them to do. Ask the viewers to complete the worksheet. Collect the worksheets and use these to guide you in follow-up teaching.

Summary

A variety of videotapes are now available on most health care subjects for patient education. Although many of these can be used effectively to teach patients, many others are unsuitable for patients with low literacy skills. To select videos that are likely to be suitable for patients with low literacy skills, give priority to videos that have a run time under 8 minutes, deal mostly with behaviors, and include interaction.

The video, by itself, cannot be relied on to teach patients. Teaching involvement is required on the part of the health care provider. Your involvement includes (1) preparations before the viewing, and (2) giving the patients a brief preview of the video, (3) assuring that there is interaction with the viewers at appropriate intervals if the 8-minute run time is exceeded.

Part 3: Teaching with Multimedia

Multimedia—What is it?

Today it means the use of sight, sound, and often interaction with a learning or entertainment system using information from stored discs or from "outside" via telephone or TV cable. For children, for whom learning to use multimedia is second nature, it means video games for entertainment or education like "Dungeons and Dragons,"© a "Sim City"© planning game, or a geography learning game like "Where in the World Is Carmen Sandiego?" For adults in industry, it is a way to be retrained to cope with a changing job market. In the health care field, it is an interactive health risk appraisal, or an interactive patient education program on diabetes management.[24]

For futurists, it is a vision of multiple sources of information accessible to an interactive learning or entertainment cubicle via the information superhighway. They see a merging of the computer with television, with on-line access to Hollywood, the library, and the university. Progress is moving to bring this vision into being, but in this chapter we present multimedia in terms of what exists today and what will be available in the very near future.

The new technology that makes interactive multimedia work is the CD-ROM (the Compact Disc–Read Only Memory) with its huge storage capacity. A single disc can store over 200,000 typed pages or 54,000 individual television picture frames—enough to store nearly all the great paintings in the world's museums.[25] The second factor that makes it work is that any picture or page on the CD-ROM can be accessed by the computer very quickly. Thus, multimedia can, within limits, imitate a real live health educator—an educator on call 24 hours a day, one who never tires, one who can instantly call up just the right illustration to explain a patient's question, one who is nonjudgmental and, in the near future, may even talk like a member of your ethnic group and in your language.

Will multimedia replace health educators? Hardly. As with all emerging technology, it can easily be oversold. One is reminded of Thomas Edison's fascination with the future of motion pictures. As late as 1925 he predicted that, "Motion picture technology will soon make books as obsolete as the horse and buggy." In fairness one must admit that television has, to some degree, accomplished that.

Still, it would be foolhardy to discount the potential impact of multimedia. Its use is growing rapidly in the schools, and is expected to make up 18 percent of corporate training budgets in 1997—up from just 2 percent in 1992.[26] In patient education, multimedia training programs are available for nutrition, diabetes, and other areas.

Availability of multimedia for patient education

The usefulness of multimedia for health educators is not seriously constrained by technology—the hardware is available—but software is limited at this writing. The software consists of computer programs built upon patient education objectives that assembles information on what is to be learned, the flowcharting of how information will be accessed, presented, and used, and the responses evaluated. The library of such programs, although growing, is still quite modest. Preliminary evidence suggests these programs can be highly suitable for people with low literacy skills.

For example, a multimedia nutrition program aimed at teaching people to choose low-cholesterol foods has been tested successfully with people in rural Appalachia.[27] The program is presented on a television screen and the viewer interacts with the TV program by means of a remote control that looks like a simple TV remote control. A TV talk show setting is used to interview a chef. He demonstrates how to make a low-cholesterol sandwich with advice from the viewer via his or her remote control. As the chef considers various foods to add to his sandwich (lettuce, mayonnaise, etc.) he asks the viewer to choose via the yes or no buttons on the remote control. Depending on the choice made by the viewer, the TV program "branches." It branches one way so the TV reinforces the good decision, or another way to show and explain what's wrong with a bad choice.

Although very few interactive programs are currently available in patient/public health education, within the next few years we can expect a rapid growth in such multimedia programs. The explosive growth of multimedia education for retraining in industry is likely to be quickly followed by a similar growth of multimedia for patient education use.

Compelling features of multimedia education are its flexibility and interaction with the learner—features that are essential for low literacy learners. For instance, it is possible to ask a question and get an answer; to highlight a word that is not understood and see an example displayed on what it means; to have any step in a process repeated as many times as needed to learn it. For health education these features are just becoming available to help patients learn. After more than 40 years of research, Bloom (1986) concluded that,

> What any person in the world can learn, almost all persons can learn if provided with appropriate prior and current conditions of learning.[28]

Multimedia appears to have the potential to provide patients with the appropriate conditions for learning. Furthermore, the patients' responses to information and questions can provide evidence that they understand the instruction—a key requirement in the new JCAHO accreditation requirements.

In summary, modern multimedia is barely here in terms of patient education, but software programs to expand its use are beginning to grow rapidly. Within the next few years, health care practitioners will be using it extensively.

References

1. Kavanagh JF (1972): Language by Ear and Eye: The Relationship Between Speech and Reading. Cambridge, MA: MIT Press, p. 135.
2. Joyce CRB, Caple G, Mason M, et al. (1969): Quantitative study of doctor-patient communication. Quarterly Journal of Medicine 38:183–194.
3. Forlizzi LA (1989): Adult Literacy in the United States Today. Institute for the Study of Adult Literacy, Penn State University, p. 4.
4. Senah CA (March 1992): Department of Health, Port of Spain, Trinidad, private correspondence.
5. Ehman J (1991): BSE Rap (tape), 199 New Scotland Ave., Albany, NY 12208.
6. Becker D (1992): Let's Pull Together: Stop Smoking Inspirational Song. Cure Heart Body Soul Program, Johns Hopkins University School of Medicine, Baltimore, MD.
7. King RC, Hill SC, Fahey LA (1979): A Report on Migrant Education Television in Australia. Australian Government Public Services, Canberra.
8. Miller GA (1956): The magical number seven. Psychol Rev 63:81.
9. Glanz K, Lewis FM, Rimer B (1991): Health Behavior and Health Education: Theory, Research and Practice. See Chapter 3, Rosentock I, The Health Belief Model: explaining behaviors through expectancies. San Francisco: Jossey Bass.

10. Walster E, Festinger L (1962): The effectiveness of "overheard" persuasive conversations. J Abnorm Psych 65(6):395–402.

11. Platt FW (1992): Conversation Failure: Case Studies in Doctor-Patient Communication. Tacoma, WA: Life Sciences Press, pp. 45–47.

12. Svarstad B, Mechanic D (1976): The Growth of Bureaucratic Medicine: An Inquiry into the Dynamics of Patient Behaviors and Organization of Medical Care. New York: John Wiley. See Chapter 11, p. 229.

13. Stitch T, Beck LJ, Hauke RN, et al. (1974): Auding and Reading: A Developmental Model. Alexandria, VA: Human Research Resources Organization. See Chapter 5.

14. Dietary Guidelines (1989): National Academy of Science, Washington, DC.

15. A whole body of literature exists on television production, but since few health care practitioners are ever tasked to produce an instructional video, the subject is not addressed in the chapter.

16. Cancer Patient Education Videotape Directory (1991): Pub. No. 91-3105. National Cancer Institute, Bethesda, MD.

17. Milner-Fenwick Video Catalog. 2125 Greenspring Drive, Timonium, MD 21093. Toll free 800/432-8433.

18. "Put Away the Frying Pan," The Health Promotion Council of Southeastern Pennsylvania, Philadelphia, PA (10-minute run time).

19. "Singing Eyes" (1994): A story about diabetes self-management. Via. Valentine, Indian Health Service Diabetes Program, Albuquerque, NM.

20. King RC, Hill SC, Fahey LA (1979): A Report on Migrant Education Television in Australia. Australian Government Public Services, Canberra.

21. Friedell GH: "For Your Peace of Mind: Get a Mammogram." The Kentucky Cancer Program, Markey Cancer Center, 800 Rose St., Lexington, KY 40536 (13-minute video).

22. "SE Met Ko"—A Video About AIDS. Haitian Women's Program, American Friends Service Committee, 15 Rutherford Place, New York, NY 10003. (In Haitian with English subtitles. Discussion guide booklet in English and Haitian.)

23. Goldman KD, Zasloff KD (1994): SOPHE News and Views: Communivision: Turning the Tables on the Media. 21(1):4, 5.

24. Health Risk Appraisal (November 1991): Healthy People Program, The Carter Center of Emory University, Atlanta, GA. Version 4.0.

25. Schwier RA, Misanchuk ER (1993): Interactive Multimedia Instruction. Englewood Cliffs, NJ: Educational Technology Publications, p. 38.

26. Washington Post (February 6, 1994).

27. Strecher V (1994): "Health Talk." An interactive video nutrition program. Health Communications Research Lab., School of Public Health, University of North Carolina, Chapel Hill, NC.

28. Bloom BS. Quoted by Trotter RJ (July 1986): The mystery of mastery. Psychology Today 20(7).

9

Tips on Teaching

"As I learned more about literacy, I began to wonder how I could identify non-readers. Then I realized that wasn't really the issue. I had to change how I presented information so that I could be sure of reaching everyone."[1]

The "Tips on Teaching" are intended to help practitioners carry out four of the steps that underlie making instructions understandable and acceptable.[2] The four steps selected are those that are particularly troublesome for teaching patients with low literacy skills. Yet they are essential if health care professionals are to avoid an information overload and to make the new information meaningful. They are also essential to cue the instructor when to review, repeat, correct, or move ahead with additional information. The four steps are:

1. Assessing what patients know about their condition or risks
2. Tying new information into what patients already know
3. Organizing meaningful feedback from patients (interaction)
4. Helping patients anticipate their experiences within the health care setting

Knowing what to expect helps people handle new experiences with greater confidence and greater motivation. With 37 million uninsured needing to access the health care system, many more poor readers new to the system are likely to come under your care.

Feedback from the patient is one element common to each of the four steps. It is this feedback that guides what you teach next, whether to stop and review or continue. Why is feedback a problem? Largely it is due to a difference in perceptions between patients and health care professionals.

151

PATIENTS	HEALTH CARE PROVIDERS
Patients may not understand that giving of information is an essential part of their health care.	Health care providers may not realize that learning is a transaction. How information is provided influences what patients learn.

Low literacy patients often lack experience in dialogue situations that deal with their personal health. In other aspects of living they have learned the hard way that the less you say the better off you are. On the other hand, many health care providers are not aware that other ways of presenting information are needed for many different types of learners.

Failure to comply with medical recommendations has several causes, but the one that health care providers can control is the way that the patient is taught. Data from recent studies by the National Council on Patient Information and Education give ample evidence of failures:[3]

PATIENT KNOWLEDGE ABOUT MEDICINES

1. Fifty percent of patients didn't know the correct dosage of their medicine.
2. Thirty-eight percent didn't know the correct timing of their doses.
3. Sixty-nine percent were not well informed about side effects.

CONSUMER ATTITUDE ABOUT MEDICINES

1. Eighty percent said they took less medicine than prescribed.
2. Seventy-two percent said they were inadequately informed about medicines.

These data indicate the need to improve the way we teach. This chapter would not be needed if the solution were only a matter of telling people information and having them deliver the answers, like pushing a button. The dilemma is that changing people's perceptions involves not only changing their knowledge, but also their attitudes, skills, and abilities.

Improving the quality of patient care includes improving the quality of the teaching. The "Tips for Teaching" are aimed at improving the **learning experiences** of patients because what patients experience is more likely to change their perceptions. Each step is discussed with the tips that will help your teaching situation whether it is a one-on-one encounter or a group session. The examples given are intended to stimulate your thinking about how to improve your teaching. Hopefully you will add your own examples as you read through the chapter.

Step 1: Assessing What Patients Know About Their Condition or Risks[4]

Finding out what the patient already knows about his condition or problem and what his attitude is toward it guides you in selecting what to teach and when to teach it. Use questions and/or devices such as pictures or cards to assess knowledge needs.

Establish the context for asking questions by saying something like, "I want to give you some information but I don't want to take up your time by telling you what you already know. So I need to ask you a few questions that will tell me what I need to teach." People need to know why they're being asked questions and what you intend to do with their responses. When they know the context, then they know how to respond.

> *Tip:* Ask questions that will give you clues such as "what" or "how" questions instead of those that can be answered with "yes" or "no." "Tell me about this problem and what you think might have caused it."

A physician told the author about a patient with a tentative diagnosis of cat scratch fever. The patient kept answering "No" to the question, "Do you have a cat?" The diagnosis was unconfirmed for several days. Finally a resident asked, "Have you ever had a cat?" At this point the patient answered, "Sure, but I gave the damn cat away after he scratched me."

In Chapter 1 the point is made about poor readers taking information literally. This case presents another example of taking a question literally.

The "what" question is useful in assessing what people think they need to learn. It is useful in different kinds of situations, i.e., for a newly diagnosed condition such as pregnancy or diabetes. The answers give you a good idea of what patients think is related to the subject and how important it is. You'll know whether to reinforce what they know, correct misinformation, or start from scratch.

- "What do you think you need to know about so that you'll have a healthy baby" (or "to keep from getting complications")?

Questions that assess patients' diet knowledge also use "what" and "how":

- "What do you think is the best way for you to cut down on eating too much fat?"
- "How do you think you can cut down on cholesterol in beef?"

> *Tip:* Use questions that pose a genuine problem for patients and that also clue you about how they currently handle the situation. ("What do you do when . . .") The answers can tell you whether to present new information, reinforce what patients are doing, or correct misinformation. Examples of these questions are shown for various situations:

- "What do you do when you run out of medicine and still feel sick?"
- "What do you do when your baby won't stop crying?"
- "When do you think that she's sick enough to call the doctor?"
- "What would you do if you woke up in the morning and found that blood had soaked through the bandage?"

Tip: Use devices such as cards, pictures, or actual equipment to identify gaps in knowledge and beliefs, and to assess the accuracy of patients' knowledge. This works well in group settings as described in the following example:

One health educator made several packs of cards with two kinds of statements about AIDS: (1) those of popular beliefs, and (2) those of scientific facts.[5] Each member of the group took a pack of cards and divided them into three piles depending on what she knew: (1) These are true. (2) These are not true. (3) I'm not sure about these. Then the health educator initiated a group discussion. Each member shared the information in each of her three piles. This information gave the staff a baseline assessment to begin the educational program.

Another approach may be useful for nutrition education. On sheets of paper or cards, paste pictures from magazines, restaurant menus, and nutrition pamphlets. Make three headings that say: "Eat all you want." "Eat if prepared right (tell how to prepare)." "Eat on your birthday." Ask the patient to sort the pictures into these categories. You will have data to give a pat on the back for the correct answers, and to review the errors in the context of presenting new and correct information.

When teaching a specific technique such as taking the baby's temperature, you want to find out what the mother(s) already know. Consider this approach:

Provide a display of two or three kinds of thermometers. Ask which one she/they would use. Rather than commenting on first responses, ask questions about where to get one, the cost, care, etc. Then continue the session, building on the information you received from the mother(s).

Assessing what patients know and believe can become a shortcut for you. It allows you to focus on critical behavioral aspects of health care and enhances motivation for the patient. It also offers an opportunity for the patient to enter into the decision making for his care and begins to develop self-efficacy.

Step 2: Tying New Information into What Patients Already Know[6,7]

The principal way that the brain "files" new information into memory is by tying it to existing knowledge (see Chapter 5, The Comprehension Process). The association of a new idea with familiar information gives meaning and logic to the new information. The challenge is to find an example that is familiar to your patients and that expresses the concept you want to get across.

Become familiar with the work and lifestyle of the patients in your rural/urban setting. Ask them to tell you about their work or their children. From their descriptions you'll obtain language cues and ways of expressing ideas that you can use later in teaching. You may even find that a part of the regimen you're teaching may not be feasible. For example, a construction worker may not be able to do urine testing for diabetes during a 10-hour shift while working on a highway job.

If you are in home health care, observe the home setting for clues to which you may have to give special thought for routine procedures. For example, how much of a problem would it be for the patient to wash her hands before and after changing a surgical dressing? Running water may not be easily available in many inner city apartments, for homeless people, and for a number of rural areas.

Tip: In teaching vocabulary select the key words, not more than three in one session, that the patient is likely to need to use in his health care.

1. Explain the meaning in the context of a sentence or two so that the patient associates the word with its meaning. For example, the word *ketones* might be critical if the patient is a diabetic. *Example:* "Ketones are chemicals that the body makes when there is not enough insulin in the blood. Ketones that build up for a long time can make you very sick and unconscious."
2. Show the word written in a pamphlet. Have the patient underline the new word and a familiar one that describes it. For example, a pamphlet describing ketones may say: "Ketones give your breath a fruity smell." (Underline *ketones* and *fruity smell.*)
3. If possible also show the word with a picture or with a synthetic body model. In the case of teaching ketones, show a picture of a person with symptoms of nausea or stomach pain so that the patient associates symptoms related to ketones with the word.
4. Ask the patient a question using the word. For example, you might say, "When do you test for ketones?" If it is appropriate, introduce a familiar word that serves as a synonym. For example, *high blood pressure* is a synonym for *hypertension.*
5. The patient needs multiple exposures to the word so that he understands it in different contexts. For example, ask how he'd explain the word to his wife (or friend). Ask him for an example of when he'd use the word. "How do I test for ketones?" If appropriate, ask when he thinks he might use the word the next time he comes to the clinic.
6. If the words lend themselves to using the actual object, such as understanding abbreviations in nutrition for amounts, use an actual teaspoon to explain "tsp." or tablespoon to explain "tbsp." In therapy situations, use pictures or synthetic models of the body, or if appropriate, the brace or device itself to explain vocabulary.

   One nurse told the author that after a visit to the OB/GYN clinic, a patient called the hospital operator and asked, "Where's your cervix?"

7. Use audiotapes to teach vocabulary. Select the key words (not more than three to start) that the patient needs to learn to manage his condition—words he'll need to use often. Make an audiotape, using the word, putting it into a sentence. Give him the tape to take home. Later have him record some sentences using the words on the tape. Eventually he can build his own word list for his condition.

Tip: Use real-life experiences to tie new information to existing knowledge. People think better when they are more relaxed and doing something. It helps relieve some of the tension and stress inherent in health care settings. Most of all, comprehension improves when the brain "exercises."

EXPERIENCING THE INSTRUCTION:

Examples follow for various situations:

Example: In one third world country a health worker planned a demonstration as part of a group session to teach how hookworm is transmitted. She had brown paper ready and asked several people to stand on the paper in their bare feet. With a felt-tip pen she drew an outline of their feet. Then she drew a dot on the foot outline to indicate where the worm could have entered their bodies.

Example: Have the patient practice the procedure and feel the benefits. For example, practicing deep breathing results in a much stronger learning experience than just being told to breathe deeply. Tell the patient: "Put your hands on your ribs and feel your own lungs fill completely with air."

Example: People need to experience the goal that they set. If weight loss is a major part of your instruction, prepare 25- or 50-pound bags of sand and have them in your office. Ask the patient to try and pick up the bag. Say: "I want you to really *feel* what you are carrying around with you. This is what you need to lose."

Example: It helps for people to taste the foods that are new to them, such as low-fat snacks. Bring the makings for low-fat snacks to a group session and have the participants make and eat them.

Example: For community workers dealing with clients in a community setting in conjunction with nutrition, invite a master gardener (available through many agricultural extension centers) to help launch a grow-it-yourself project. Initiate a community garden program under the guidance of a master gardener consultant. Have a harvest fair or harvest supper at the end of the season to celebrate the successful gardens.

SIMULATING THE INSTRUCTION:

Examples follow for various situations:

Example: There are different ways to obtain information about dietary habits. Instead of using a questionnaire, consider obtaining your information by using a simulation experience. Create a cafeteria line using food models and ask people to select what they usually eat for breakfast, lunch, and dinner. The results may not be as accurate as you wish, but the opportunities to clarify information are much greater than if you rely only on oral responses.

Example: In teaching nutrition, create a grocery store setting where clients can learn to read ingredient labels, select foods for a prescribed diet, use unit-pricing information, and do comparison shopping for store brands versus advertised brands. This could also be an exhibit in the waiting room.

Example: Video is particularly well adapted to help simulate health care experiences. For surgical procedures or different forms of therapy, video offers the motion as well as the visual image to help the patient anticipate the experience (see Chapter 8, Teaching with Technology). It is important for learning to provide opportunity for the patient to respond and ask questions.

Example: Play equipment can be used for adults as well as children. For example, when the author used play equipment in the dental clinic, adults as well as children became very interested in going through the experience of making fillings and placing them in the teeth. The experience of working directly with the things the dentist would use later gave them a sense of confidence that it wasn't going to be "too bad."

To teach when to take medicine, consider using a sheet such as Figure 9-1. If the patient can mark the hands on the clocks for the appropriate times, and draw circles around the pictures of the medicines, it will create more interest and help memory.

Tip: Review and reinforce new information. People need to have new information reviewed often so that it can be firmly tied to their existing knowledge. Plan for variety in the ways that you review and reinforce. In this way you are able to achieve a better match with the learning styles of different people. Some of us are visual learners, some auditory, some tactile. Here are some ways to review new information and at the same time introduce variety in your teaching:

For a specific procedure: Prepare cards with each step of the procedure pictured on a single card. Ask the patient to put the cards in a row, in the order for carrying out the procedure correctly.

FIGURE 9-1

Reminder sheet for medications that the patient marks and takes home. *(Source:* Do You Understand? Literacy Volunteers of America, 5795 Widewaters Parkway, Syracuse, NY 13214-1836)

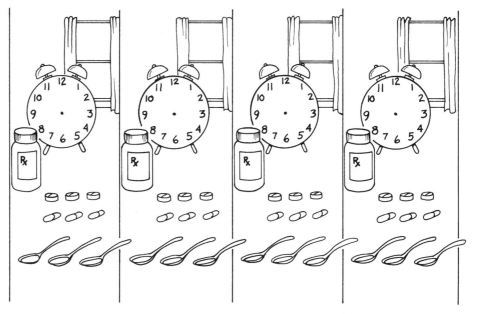

For behavior change: To encourage patients to quit smoking, make a pack of cards with a few words (or pictures) on each, suggesting things they could do when they get the urge to smoke—take a walk, call a friend, eat an apple, go fishing, etc. Have the patients sort the cards with those activities most likely to be chosen on top, those least likely on the bottom.

As a reminder: "Five-Finger Reminder": Draw the patient's hand on an 8½-by-11-inch piece of paper. On each finger and the thumb, write the things the patient suggests she can do to keep from getting angry at her children. Put it on the refrigerator door.

Low literacy patients may well have to hear information more than once. They need to practice what they're supposed to do in small steps several times. When the patient is practicing and begins to struggle, suggest two possibilities. Ask the patient to choose the one he thinks is the best. If that doesn't work, give the correct response; then come back later to give the patient the chance to succeed.

For both review and reinforcement, consider using a videotape or an audiotape on the subject. Afterward, discuss what the patients found out that they didn't know before or hadn't thought about. Use low-reading-level pamphlets that they can take home and share with their friends or family.

If the purpose is suitable, plan on using a demonstration for review. Have the patient show how to carry out the procedure. For a diabetes class, one diabetes educator told the group that next week they would review foot care by having everyone take off their shoes and stockings and they would examine each other's feet.

They came prepared for the session, and to the instructor's surprise, they were much more thorough in making their examinations than she thought possible.

Consider the following examples for reinforcement:

- If you're advising a midday rest, hand out a "Couch Potato License" with rest hours listed on it.
- For patients who need to watch their diet, with their help, make a refrigerator calendar of "Snack of the Day."
- Have a selection of recipes and have patients copy three new recipes they agree to try. Give them a return postcard with check-off boxes to tell what they thought of them.

Step 3: Organize Meaningful Feedback from Patients (Interaction)[8]

Tip: Plan a portion of your instruction for feedback from the patient. One way to organize feedback is to plan to use at least the last few minutes of an instruction for a rehearsal speech by the patient on how she'll explain what she has just learned to her family. If you have several patients in the same circumstance, have them work in pairs and explain what they've just learned to one another. The instructor should monitor these interactions. Later, have them share what they have learned with the whole group.

Include a family member in this initial instruction if possible. If two people get the information, they can check with each other later on the accuracy of their memories. Furthermore, they reinforce one another.

Review written material together; when you ask the patient to underline the most important information, it shows that you care about her learning. Interaction of this kind serves to stimulate memory.

Even a pamphlet with a high reading level can be used by marking off ahead of time the particular page or visual that you want the patient to have. In this way the patient will not be intimidated by going through the material just to find one page that is useful.

Teach patients in pairs so they can share the learning experience and reinforce each other. The more patients can rehearse and see the application of new information to their real-life situation, the greater the chances for long-term memory retention and compliance. This kind of sharing can work well with patients of a mixed socioeconomic background and with a mix of reading skill levels. The reason it works is that the sharing session is problem centered rather than subject centered. People are more willing to share when they perceive that they have common problems. They're "all in the same boat."

> *Tip:* Summarize what the patient is to do. Another way to organize feedback is to summarize what the patient is to do using an easy-to-read handout sheet or pamphlet. This sheet is then given to the patient to take home. For example, after the tests are completed and the health care provider is ready to dispense medicines or write a prescription, take your time to explain carefully how each medication is intended to help. Point to the medication listed on the written handout.

Ask the patient what it is for. Then explain the dosage and again use the sheet to make sure the patient knows where it is written down. Tell the side effects and show where they are explained on the sheet. Then the health care provider might say:

"I want to be sure I didn't leave anything out that I should have told you. Would you tell me now what you are to do so that I can be sure you know what is important? You can use this handout sheet as you tell me what medicines you will take and when you'll take them, the dosage, etc. What about diet? Exercise? Rest?"

> *Tip:* Plan with the patient to recognize small successes. Because many poor readers suffer from low self-esteem they need to feel good about the effort they make. You can help them to feel good. Plan the health education session so that they can experience small successes along the way. Giving them support by saying, "You're right!" may be sufficient. However, there are additional ways to reward small successes. Here are some examples:

Example: Together with the patient, make a list of nonfood rewards for days when the patient completes an exercise routine, keeps a diet plan, stays off cigarettes, or doesn't yell at the kids.

Example: Color Me Healthy": Have waiting room coloring sheets on a variety of subjects or that show traditional foods for holidays.

Example: "Health Hero/Heroine of the Month": Use an overhead projector or other light source to project a strong light on a poster board. Have the person sit between the light and the board to create a silhouette. Draw around the shadow. Caption the picture with the accomplishment (e.g., quit smoking, lowered cholesterol, had kids immunized). Print the name of the honoree. Change every month.

Example: Some weeks after surgery, the moment arrives to suggest or reinforce lifestyle changes that will lower the risk of recurrence or complications. Sending patients an easy-to-read pamphlet or newsletter may be just the trigger needed to initiate the desired behavior. We can all use a gentle prod, but low literacy patients may especially benefit from verbal and pictorial information about how to access exercise programs, support groups, or other resources. They do not regularly read a newspaper or see notices that come to the attention of more skilled readers.

Step 4: Helping Patients Anticipate Their Experiences Within the Health Care Setting[9]

Preparing people for what is likely to happen makes the experience less traumatic and therefore more manageable. The health care setting is not intimidating to us because we know what to expect. However, it can create anxiety for people without good reading skills who lack a fluent vocabulary for making themselves understood. Once they are within "the system" they might think they would be bothering the nurse or doctor if they asked questions. They don't want to be perceived as making a fuss. If they are from a different culture, the experience can be more intimidating.

> *Tip:* Provide orientation to patients on what to expect within the health care setting. Patients need to understand and be able to anticipate the experience they will have in the hospital or clinic system. Orientation can be provided in different ways by staff and also by trained volunteers from the community. Five tips on what the orientation might include are given below:

1. Patients must answer many questions: Many patients are not prepared for this. It would help to be told in advance:

"You will be asked a lot of questions from the time you arrive until you leave. You will be asked about your name, where you live, your family, as well as about your illness or reason for being there. Doctors, nurses, and other people ask you questions because they have a lot of different ways they can help you. They have to select the way that is best for you."

Without this kind of explanation, patients can get a completely wrong impression. The author was told by one patient, "He can't be a very good doctor if he has to ask so many questions." Patients might be told:

"It is the information that you give the doctors that helps them pick the treatment that is best for you. So if you don't understand their question, be sure to tell them that you don't understand. They'll be glad to explain it. Your information is most important.

"Sometimes you will be asked the same question by different people. That's okay. All staff members have to keep their own records so that they can use the information for the special way that they can help you best.

"On return visits, you will be asked questions again. Doctors and nurses need to know whether to keep you on the same treatment or whether to change it. So they ask questions to help make the treatment right for you."

2. To explain receiving treatment from different professionals, the patient might be told:

"You may need to see different doctors or nurses or others who have special training for your particular problem. They have many different ways to help you. They want to be sure that you get what you need.

"Doctors and nurses and other staff all have a work schedule that they have to follow. The doctor that sees you the first time may not be working on the day when you come back. So you may see a different one depending on the work schedule or the kind of help you need. It may take a little longer if you have a different doctor but don't worry about it. The doctors and nurses will be using your record that you helped with when you answered all those questions."

3. You can legitimatize the asking of questions about words patients don't understand by saying something like this:

"It's not only okay but doctors and nurses want you to ask questions when you don't understand the words they're using. They use big words so much in talking to other professionals that they may forget you do not know those words. Ask them to give you an example of what they're explaining, or show you a picture of it.

"Sometimes doctors and nurses use words you are familiar with but they have a different meaning in health care. For example, they may talk about your body "cells." You may think they're talking about a "jail cell." They're talking about the very small parts of your body. The word cell has a different meaning here.

"If what they're telling you doesn't make sense to you, ask them to stop and explain the word. Don't be afraid to tell them what you think the word means. They have no way of knowing unless you tell them. You will be helping them by letting them know that you don't understand.

"They can use pictures, show you, or call in another person who can help you. Don't guess or think that you'll ask your friends to help you. Most of the time they won't know either. It saves time if you let the doctor and nurse know right away."

4. To help patients understand that results from lab tests may take days or longer, say:

"It may take several days or several weeks for doctors and nurses to learn the results of your tests. This is because several other people have to take part in the testing process. And those people may have to wait a few days, too, if there is some special test they have to carry out. Sometimes your test may need to be seen by people in other cities or other clinics so they can give your doctor and nurse the best information.

"Doctors and nurses also wish that you could get the answers faster. But new tests have many steps and they each take a certain amount of time."

5. To help patients understand that appointments for follow-up are just as important as their first visit, you might say:

"Depending on what's wrong with you, you may be asked to return so the doctors and nurses and others can see how well you are doing. This happens all the time to almost everybody. It's because we all respond differently to treatment. You may need a different medicine, or treatment. It is very important for you to return to see the doctors and nurses when they tell you to. They may give you a piece of paper called an appointment slip with the date and time marked on it.

"You may be asked to see other people who have special training such as people to help you walk or talk better. This kind of help is called rehabilitation. Sometimes it may not be clear to you why you are being asked to see them."

Most institutions have a pamphlet or a means to orient patients to the particular care they may receive, e.g., pregnancy, checkups, surgery, rehabilitation. The above scenarios explain some of the "culture" of the health care system to people who don't have the logic, language, or experience skills to have learned this procedural information on their own.

Additional Tips

Handling information that you didn't have time to teach: When you want to keep the amount of information within your time limits or the patient's, consider using other media. The patient can take the information home to review under less stressful conditions. You might say:

"There are other things you should know that will help you in your recovery. I've made an audiotape you can play when you get home that will tell you about some of these things. I will call you in a day or two and we can go over any questions that you have." (Most people, including those with low literacy skills, have tape recorders or have easy access to one.)

If you find yourself approaching burnout from repeating the same instructions, an audiotape or videotape can be an ever-patient teacher. If you have taught a concept in your traditional way and there are patients who need review, use a different medium for a second (or third) instruction.

Check out your media carefully—use SAM (see Chapter 4, Assessing Suitability of Materials), a materials checklist, or a group of patients to review for the suitability of any medium you use.

Coping with distractions: Distractions are a frequent concern in all health agency settings. They may come from children wanting attention, telephones, radios, TVs, or construction and street noise. The patient may also be preoccupied by stress or for other reasons that you can't detect.

Don't try to talk through the distractions. If you do not have the patient's attention, wait until you do. If it is not forthcoming, you might say, "This does not seem to be a good time for us to talk. Tell me when it would be better for you because this is important." This approach opens up the topic of why it's important and the need to enlist cooperation from the patient. It is common for people with low literacy skills to have multiple problems.

Children in the home or who accompany parents to other settings can make concentration impossible for adults. Try to engage the children in other activities or provide space for youngsters apart from their parents, if you can.

Two Case Studies: Putting It All Together

Two case studies are presented that apply many of the points made earlier in this chapter. The first case study is for a one-on-one interaction and the second case study is for group teaching.

Case 1: One-on-one interaction: building an agenda to increase compliance

One of the most common interactions between health care providers and patients occurs when a diagnosis has been made and a prescription for care is advised.

Ley and colleagues have shown that organizing what is said into an agenda and following a logical sequence can increase recall nearly 50 percent.[10] Such a conversation begins by telling a patient what the agenda contains: *"I'm going to tell you:*

1. What I think is wrong with you.
2. What tests we need to carry out to be sure.
3. What I think will happen to you.
4. What treatment you will need.
5. What you can do to help yourself."

Then each point is "fleshed out" with appropriate information:

Probable diagnosis: "You have a chest infection. Your larynx is slightly inflamed. But I think your heart is all right."

Tests needed: "We will do some tests to make sure. We will need to take a blood sample and a chest x-ray."

Outcome prediction: "Your cough should disappear in the next two days. You will feel better in a week or so, and you should recover completely."

What I can do: "I will give you an injection of an antibiotic and some pills to take for 10 days. I will give you an inhaler to use when you get stuffed up and can't breathe."

What you can do: "You should keep out of cold drafts and stay inside when the weather is foggy. It would be good to get two hours of rest every afternoon. If you continue to feel sick after three or four days, call me."

By framing the information in this way, the advance organizers signal where the conversation is going. The patient is able to gather the threads of information with ease and is much more likely to remember them. health care providers are much less likely to leave out steps important to the patient if they adopt an agenda approach to their instruction.

Case 2: Group teaching: sharing the information[11,12]

Effective group teaching is highly participatory and open in the sense that group members respond to questions rather than a didactic or more closed teacher-student interaction. This shared-response approach builds group cohesion, which aids motivation. Even responses that miss the point are welcome. They help clear up misconceptions and provide opportunities to make critical judgments. These are essential to self-confidence in managing a situation.

A basic agenda may look like this:

Preparation: Plan to review information from the previous session in an interactive way. For example, to review a session on bathing and dressing a baby, show the participants a series of pictures that illustrate good practice. Ask them to explain why the action shown is important.

Arrive early enough to check on the facilities. Greet each person upon arrival. This sets the tone for the session and invites interchanges that might be appropriate for the session.

Objective: Present a brief outline of what is to be learned at the session. For example: "Today we will learn how to take your baby's temperature and what to do if your baby has a fever."

The Session:
1. Begin by exploring what the clients already know (Step 1 in this chapter). For example, provide a display of two or three kinds of thermometers. Ask which one they would use to take a baby's temperature. Rather than commenting on first responses, encourage others to answer.
2. Lead a brief discussion (not a lecture) asking questions about what makes the correct thermometer appropriate. Then talk about where to get one, the cost, care, etc.
3. Using a baby or doll model, if you have one, demonstrate the correct procedure. Clients need to see the action and see themselves doing it. Talk your way through the action while you demonstrate.
4. Ask the clients to follow your example and tell what steps they are taking while they practice. If they feel uncomfortable doing this, explain that it is a memory aid and will really make a difference in what they learn and how they do it.
5. Continue with a discussion of other aspects of what to do if you think your baby has a fever.

Review and verification:

1. Provide a way to check on each important point. For example, have group members read thermometers with different temperatures displayed.
2. Review all major points. *Example:* Give pairs of participants descriptions of different situations. One possible situation might be, "Your mother-in-law says, 'You don't need to take the baby's temperature. Just feel his forehead.' Ask, "What are the steps you would take to deal with this situation?" After you give an example, ask the participants for examples of other situations where they might need to explain why they're taking the baby's temperature.
3. Provide easy-to-read materials and pictures that review the points made in the session just completed. Write each participant's name on the copy you hand out to them. That sends the message, "This is meant for you!" Point out where the key information is located as a further review. Have participants use a colored marker to highlight the important points.

Getting ready for the next session:

1. Give a preview of the next session. This could be a brief skit for the next session that indicates the topic to be discussed. For example, "A new mother picks up the phone as she says, 'I wonder what Mary does when Jason won't stop crying.'" This should raise questions but give no answers—a teaser to encourage clients to return.
2. Thank each participant, and if you feel inclined, add a personal remark. For example, "You gave us some good examples today. Thanks!" Or to a quiet person, "I'm glad you could join us today."

Instructors often ask about how to handle different kinds of personalities and learning styles in group sessions. Table 9-1 identifies six kinds of problems you may encounter and some possible ways of handling them.

TABLE 9-1

Ways to improve effectiveness in group instruction

PROBLEMS	POSSIBLE SOLUTIONS
1. Anxiety high for the less skilled.	1. Don't call on individuals. Ask them to work in pairs.
2. Wide learning differences and learning styles.	2. Use video, audio, pictures, in repeated presentations.
3. Some participants are slow to learn.	3. Teach in small units; review often; provide repeated examples and practice times.
4. Quick learners may become bored.	4. Ask them to demonstrate and teach others; use variety of teaching methods.
5. Feedback is hesitant and uncertain.	5. Clarify success criteria; ask participants to self-evaluate in pairs.
6. Record keeping is difficult.	6. Make a clear teaching plan; use checklists to monitor progress.

Summary

Improving teaching methods requires a willingness to reach out and try new ways of communicating with patients or clients. People remember better when they find things out for themselves and have the opportunity to apply what they have learned. Organizing a teaching plan ahead of time makes it possible to be sure you've included the key points. Sharing the agenda with the patients helps them remember your message.

Experiencing the information is the most likely way to accept and remember it. Teaching in a family or in a group situation creates opportunities for broader experiences to be brought to bear on the problems. In the American culture the teacher is not the sine qua non of information but rather the facilitator of learning for others.

References

1. Szudy E, Arroyo MG (1994): The Right to Understand: Linking Literacy to Health and Safety Training. Berkeley, CA: Labor Occupational Health Program, University of California at Berkeley. See Chapter 3, Getting to know your audience, p. 37.
2. These tips help in meeting new patient education standards. Accreditation Manual for Hospitals (1993): Patient and Family Education. Joint Commission on Accreditation of Healthcare Organizations, One Renaissance Blvd., Oakbrook Terrace, IL 60181.
3. Compliance: Do the Right Thing—A Planning Guide (October 1992): National Council of Patient Information and Education, 666 11th St. NW, Suite 810, Washington, DC 20001.
4. Knowles, M (1978): The Adult Learner: A Neglected Species. Houston, TX: Gulf Publishing Co. See Chapter 3, A theory of adult learning: andragogy.
5. Ramos L. MPH Project Manager. Latinas AIDS Literacy Project, University of Southern California Department of Family Medicine, 1420 San Pablo St., PMB-B205, Los Angeles, CA 90033.
6. Werner D, Bower B (1982): Starting with What Is Already Familiar to Students. Helping Health Workers Learn (Chapters 5–11). The Hesperian Foundation, PO Box 1692, Palo Alto, CA 94302.
7. Thelen JN (April 1986): Vocabulary instruction and meaningful learning. Journal of Reading 29(7):603–609.
8. Hand JD (1982): Brain functions during learning: implications for text design. As contained in DH Jonassen (ed), The Technology of Text: Principles for Structuring, Designing, and Displaying Text. Englewood Cliffs, NJ: Educational Technology Publications.
9. Bandura A (1977): How individuals, environments, and health behavior interact: social learning theory. As contained in K Glanz, FM Lewis, and BK Rimer (eds), Health Behavior and Health Education: Theory, Research and Practice. San Francisco: Jossey-Bass.
10. Ley P, Eaves D, Walker, CM (1973): A method for increasing patients' recall of information presented by doctors. Psychological Medicine 3:217.
11. Werner D, Bower B (1982): Helping Health Workers Learn. Hesperian Foundation, PO Box 1692, Palo Alto, CA 94302. See Chapter 5: Planning a class, pp.5-1—5-18.
12. Cartwright D, Zander, A (1968): Group Dynamics: Research and Theory, 3rd ed. New York: Harper & Row, 580p.

10

"How do I find out if patients can understand the material?"

Learner Verification and Revision of Materials

The Concept

Learner verification and revision[1] is an interview procedure to verify the suitability of a health instruction with the population who is to use it. The purpose is to assure that mismatches in communication as well as unsuitable design and content are uncovered. Learner verification and revision is especially useful during the development phase. For materials already completed, it can reveal the need for supplemental teaching aids.

Since it is formative research, only small samples are required. The procedure is not time-consuming and can be conducted within normal work schedules. Objectives for the reader of this chapter are:

1. To learn how to carry out the learner verification procedure
2. To evaluate its results

The Rationale

Because of the training and experience of health care professionals, they do not share the same logic, language, and experience as the rest of the American population. Thus, there are often mismatches and gaps in the instructions. For the intended population, these communication problems may lead to misunderstanding, disbelief, and rejection of the health instruction. Learner verification and revision uncovers the specific content or format features of an instruction that are not understood or accepted, and the process often produces remedies.

167

Here are a few simple examples of how we "talk by" each other:

- One of the authors tested the word "avoid" in a nutrition pamphlet with eleven patients in a metropolitan hospital (1992). Only one of the eleven knew the behavior for "avoid".
- Nutrition claims in advertisments are often misinterpreted. For example, the term "cholesterol-lowering" was often mistaken to mean "low calorie".[2]
- For quite some time we've known that patient knowledge of medical vocabulary is poor. Words like "cardiac, orally, therapy" were understood by less than 50% of those tested (Samora, 1960).[3] Similar work by Larrabee (1977) continued to show problems with words such as "palpitations, stroke, sputum, thyroid" etc.[4]

Quality assurance of educational materials is essential to achieve patient education program objectives. Learner verification and revision is a process that improves quality by finding out what people understand from an instruction while it is still in draft form and easy to change.

Some comments from health care professionals who have found Learner Verification and Revision to be highly useful are as follows:

- "It is so easy to do. I take my draft and go visit 5 or 10 patients. It's amazing what they see in the instructions that I would never see."[5]
- "These interview techniques (qualitative) were found to be quite satisfactory in eliciting expression of beliefs, feelings, and attitudes about the nutrition materials being tested."[6]
- "The assessment identified portions of text and graphics that confused some readers. We used that assessment to improve the booklets by changing the confusing text and illustrations."[7]
- "After testing four drafts of a cover for our booklet, we took a hard look at our objective. It was to inform patients about a procedure. . . Then the rest was easy."[8]

Specific Elements to Be Verified

Learner verification and revision identifies the likelihood of the instruction influencing its audience: Will it be attractive to the audience? Can people understand it? Do they feel that they can carry out the message? Is it culturally suitable? Does it make sense to carry out the message?

Attraction: First the communication needs to attract its audience. If the patient doesn't look at it, there's no chance for influence. Is the instruction appealing enough to carry the patient into the message itself? Are the visuals of interest? Do the colors fit the tone and mood of the subject? For an audiotape or videotape, is the voice easy to listen to? Is the diction distinct? Is the speed reasonable? Is the accent understandable? Are any aids needed?

Comprehension: This is a critical component for all patients. It is especially critical for patients with low literacy skills because they can access fewer information resources than highly literate patients. Can the patients tell you in their own words what the message meant? What other interpretations are possible?

Are there so many actions asked for that the patients become confused? Are there concept, category, or value judgment words used that may not mean to patients what they mean to you?

Can the patients demonstrate, show you, or tell you what they believe they are supposed to do as a result of being exposed to your message? Comprehension occurs when the person can convert the message from one format to another. So if patients look or listen they should be able to restate the message by demonstrating or showing you what the message says.

Self-efficacy: Do patients feel that the message is doable for them? Do they feel confident that they have enough information and skill to carry out the instruction? If they are uncertain, what kind of additional instruction is needed?

Cultural acceptability: Is the message in any way offensive? Is the message perceived as true? Are there any annoying elements? Hair styles, jewelry, dress, and background settings all enhance or detract from cultural suitability. The ways that deeper aspects of culture may be presented or alluded to also strongly influence cultural acceptance. Such aspects include child-rearing practices, roles of men and women, views about birth and death.

Persuasion: Is the message able to convince people that they should take action? Would other people in the community likely follow this advice? What might this instruction say that would make it more helpful?

Learner Verification and Revision Procedure: The Overview

What kinds of media can be verified? All media can be verified. When do you verify? At the conceptual stage, draft stages, or upon completion. The most cost-effective time is in the concept or early draft stage.

Step 1: Preparation

DETERMINE THE OBJECTIVE (PURPOSE) OF THE MATERIAL

Since few instructions state the objective, you may need to study the instruction and ask yourself, What should the person be able to do after reading, viewing, or listening? Write out your perception of what the instruction should accomplish.

Identify the key points of the message and the likely trouble spots. Write down the key points that you think are critical for the patients to understand in order to carry out the message or behaviors. The key points may be located up front, in the middle, or at the end. Likely trouble spots include the meaning of any concept, category, or value judgment words. What parts of the visuals need testing? Will the layout be easy or hard for poor readers? Trouble spots also include typography. The key points and likely trouble spots are a critical input to the next step.

PREPARE THE QUESTIONS FOR THE INTERVIEW

Questions need to test patients' understanding of the key points mentioned above. Questions also need to determine the likely influence of the instructions, i.e., attraction, self-efficacy, cultural acceptability, and persuasion.

Train interviewers

A short orientation for interviewers may be needed to help them understand that learner verification and revision is *not* an instructional session. The purpose is to obtain feedback on how well people understand the information presented. The learner verification and revision process is not difficult—it's fascinating—and it is not time-consuming.

Plan the sample and select test sites

Plan the sample to include the age and gender according to the nature of the message. The size of the sample depends on the level of confidence you want; for national distribution of the material use a sample size of 30–50. For local use, a sample size of 10 may be sufficient. Select test sites where the intended audience is likely to be found.

Step 2: Interview respondents (patients)

During most learner verification and revision interviews respondents are asked to retain the material and are encouraged to refer to it throughout the interview. Follow the sequence of questions in the order they are written on the questionnaire. Record responses verbatim. Do not ad lib or interrupt the respondents. If the respondent is tired or wants to quit, fine. Mark the interview incomplete and proceed to the next person. Typically the interview takes about 15–20 minutes.

Step 3: Evaluate responses and revise

Tabulate the responses to the questions and look for answers that are different from what you expected. Evaluate the differences by asking yourself, How important are they in terms of the patient carrying out the message? Is this misunderstanding going to cause real problems? Or is it nice to know but not essential? How many patients had the same number of different or incorrect responses?

Revise according to the nature of the trouble spots and the number of patients who gave incorrect responses. Retest to make sure that any major revisions have indeed corrected the trouble spots and not introduced new ones.

This completes the overview of the learner verification and review procedure. Detailed information is now given for each of the steps, along with examples.

Learner Verification and Revision: The Details

Step 1: Preparation

The objective of the material

Sometimes this task is easy because the objective is clearly stated in the title in easy-to-understand language. However, sometimes you may have to study the material to decide on the objective.

FIGURE 10-1

Poster on nutrition for cancer prevention. Objective of message: to motivate people to eat five fruits and vegetables every day. (*Source:* National Cancer Institute, Branch of Special Populations, Nutrition Project, draft poster, 1992)

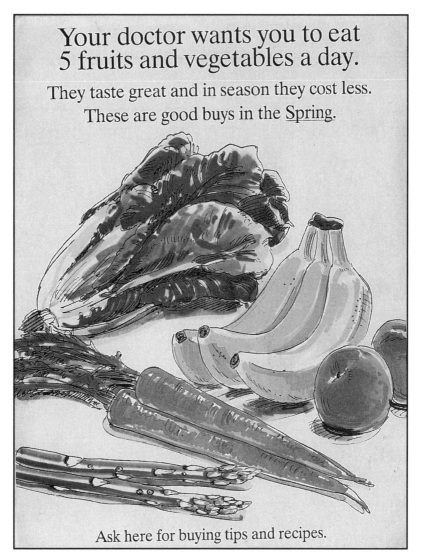

Objectives can be stated in different terms, i.e., behavior, motivation, or knowledge. The substance of the testing flows from the objectives (purpose). The objectives also serve as a guide in the evaluation of what should be revised when the responses have been compiled. Save yourself considerable time and effort by having as clear and accurate a statement of objectives as possible. So that you might see how much objectives can differ, two examples are shown. Figure 10-1 is a nutrition poster for motivational purposes.

Figures 10-2 through 10-5 show a typical threefold pamphlet. The cover gives the subject, osteoporosis; the inside folded page tells you where you can be tested; and the back cover gives the name of the medical institution: Queens Medical Center. The educational objectives of this pamphlet are to (1) create an awareness of the seriousness of osteoporosis among women at risk; (2) tell what the patient can do to cut her risk of getting osteoporosis; (3) motivate her to take action.

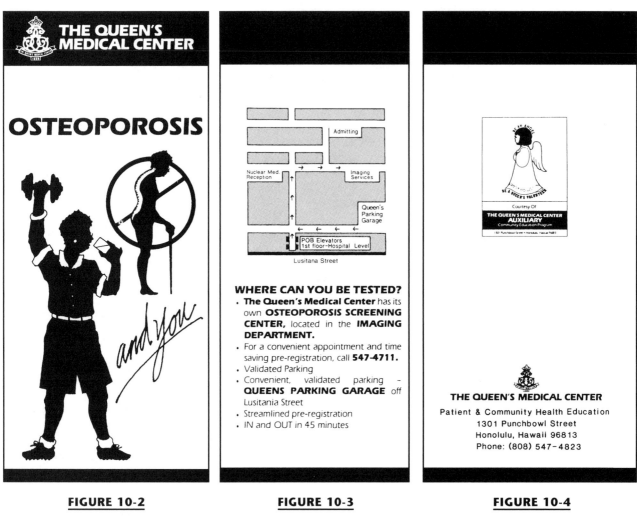

FIGURE 10-2

Front cover. (*Source:* Osteoporosis and You. Queens Medical Center, Honolulu, HI)

FIGURE 10-3

Inside fold.

FIGURE 10-4

Back cover.

Key points and likely trouble spots

Include on your list of key points only those essential to carrying out the objectives of the material. Not every sentence or every piece of artwork needs to be tested. By identifying the key points you are singling out those parts of the material that need to be tested (perhaps three or four key points that explain the objectives). Give priority to the actions or behaviors the patient needs to carry out. These are examples of key points:

1. FIGURE 10-1: poster on nutrition for cancer prevention:
   —Your doctor wants you to eat five fruits and vegetables every day.
   —Identify fruits and vegetables pictured.
   —Fruits and vegetables taste great; they cost less in season.

WHAT IS OSTEOPOROSIS?

OSTEOPOROSIS is a condition in which there is thinning of the bones because of loss of calcium. This increases the risk of breaking bones of the spine, wrist and hip areas. It is often recognized by a curving of the upper spine, commonly known as "hunch back."

- One out of every four American women is affected by it.
- **80%** of people with broken hips have **OSTEOPOROSIS.**
- **20%** of these people will **die** from complications within three months.
- It is a **SILENT DISEASE** because it is not discovered until a broken bone occurs.
- It **CANNOT** be **TREATED**, but it **CAN** be **PREVENTED** if calcium loss is found early.

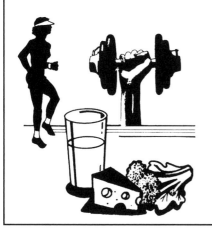

WHAT ARE THE RISK FACTORS FOR OSTEOPOROSIS?

RISK FACTORS THAT YOU CAN CHANGE

- **NUTRITIONAL FACTORS**
  - Calcium Deficiency
  - Vitamin D Deficiency
- **BONE ROBBING HABITS**
  - Too much caffeine
  - High protein diet
  - High fiber foods
  - Too much salt
  - Too much alcohol
  - Physical inactivity
  - Smoking

RISK FACTORS THAT YOU CANNOT CHANGE

- **RACE** (Caucasians and Orientals are more prone to get osteoporosis)
- **FAMILY HISTORY** of Osteoporosis
- **MENOPAUSE**
- **SMALL, FINE BONES**
- **ALLERGY** to milk and milk products

HOW IS IT FOUND?

OSTEOPOROSIS can be identified through a simple and painless **bone density scan** (photon absorptimetry).

- This test can show as little as 1% bone loss.
- It takes less than 30 minutes for the scanning process.

Regular x-rays can detect osteoporosis, but only in its **ADVANCED STAGES.**

HOW CAN YOU PREVENT OSTEOPOROSIS?

- Eat a balanced diet from each of the four food groups:
  - milk
  - meat, poultry and fish
  - vegetables and fruits
  - breads and cereals
- Reduce your intake of alcohol and caffeine.
- Stop smoking.
- Exercise regularly. Do weight-bearing exercises such as running, walking, jogging, bicycling or hiking.
- Avoid stress.
- Ask your doctor about ESTROGEN REPLACEMENT THERAPY (ERT).
- Make sure you get enough calcium and Vitamin D.
  - Eat foods rich in calcium, such as:

FOOD	MEASURE	CALCIUM CONTENT
Beans – canned	1 cup	138-159
Broccoli – cooked	1 cup	136
Cabbage – cooked	1 cup	140
Cheese – cheddar	1 oz.	213
cottage	1 cup	212
Ice Cream	1 cup	194
Milk – skim	1 cup	296
Salmon – canned	½ cup	170
Sardines – canned	2 oz.	261
Taro leaves – cooked	1 cup	178
Tofu	¼ block	252
Turnip greens	1 cup	267
Yogurt	1 cup	272

FIGURE 10-5

Most of the content is in the centerfold, which addresses osteoporosis, the risks, and how to prevent it.

2. **FIGURES 10-2** through **10-5**: a threefold pamphlet on osteoporosis:
   —Understanding what osteoporosis is.
   —Identifying risk factors you can change.
   —Understanding what to do to prevent osteoporosis.
   —Knowing how to detect it.

ARE CERTAIN WORDS LIKELY TO CAUSE PROBLEMS?

To identify potential trouble spots, look for words, phrases, and illustrations that must be understood if the reader/viewer is to get the key points you've written out. For example, if a key point is about diet, include a question to ask what the word tells you to do. For many people it means a two-week semi-starvation period. To a nutritionist it may mean a lifelong meal plan.

Words that express a concept, category, or value judgment are potential trouble spots (see Chapter 6 for examples). They may not be perceived by patients in the same way that you perceive them. Examples of the kinds of questions that can be asked to determine understanding are given in Table 10-1. The purpose of the question or the reason for it are given on the left side and the sample questions are on the right side.

WILL THE ARTWORK (VISUALS, GRAPHICS) HELP OR CONFUSE THE KEY POINTS?

Artwork needs to be tested. Consider the following sample questions (as relevant for the particular material):

- Let's look at the cover. What catches your eye?
- What do the pictures tell you?
- What do you think of the color?

LAYOUT: DOES THE READER HAVE TO LOOK IN SEVERAL DIRECTIONS TO FOLLOW THE MESSAGE?

Poor layout can create comprehension problems. For example, going to one part of the page for one piece of information, then moving up or down the page like tic-tac-toe to get to the next point is hard for poor readers. They lose their place and may decide to quit (see Chapter 7).

Questions for the interview

Use open-ended questions, i.e., "what," "where," "when," "how," and "why" questions instead of questions requiring answers of "yes" or "no." These questions are best for identifying the specific trouble spots in the instruction. Establish a neutral tone to eliminate bias:

- *Neutral question:* Do these people look like anyone you know?
- *Biased question:* Don't you think these are good pictures?

TABLE 10-1

Examples of different kinds of questions to determine understanding of commonly used words and phrases in health care instructions

PURPOSE FOR THE QUESTION	EXAMPLE OF QUESTIONS (FROM DIFFERENT KINDS OF INSTRUCTIONS)
Testing individual words	1. The word *avoid* means different things to different people. What does the word tell you to do?
Obtain an example to determine understanding of the context of the word	2. What does the pamphlet mean when it says to eat balanced meals? For instance, what would you eat for lunch to have a balanced meal?
Distinguishing key details	3. What do these numbers for blood pressure tell you?
Ask for behavior information when testing a list of signs and symptoms	4. What kind of things might go wrong with the baby that would tell you to take the baby to the doctor?

HOW MANY QUESTIONS SHOULD YOU ASK?

For short pamphlets, posters, videotapes, and audiotapes a total of about 10–15 questions should be sufficient. For longer material, try to limit the total to about 20 questions.

WHICH QUESTIONS SHOULD YOU ASK FIRST?

Begin with an open-ended question about comprehension. Use this or a similar question: "Tell me in your own words, what is this all about?" You want to find out if the respondent has the sense of the instruction. It is important to know if the person is able to tell you the main theme or purpose of the instruction. This is as important as the details.

DESIGN OF SPECIFIC TYPES OF QUESTIONS

- SELF-EFFICACY: Questions that ask, "Tell me, how and when would you do this?" or "Would you need to know anything else before doing this?" are very useful in getting a sense of the person's confidence with the instruction. It also enables you to know what additional help or information needs to be added.
- CULTURAL ACCEPTABILITY: To help bring out any different perceptions of what is being shown use a question such as, "Is this _____ okay for showing a family like yours? (or friends of yours?). Then follow with a question such as, "What might be a better way to show _____?
- PERSUASION: Questions such as, "Do you think your friends and neighbors would be willing to try this?" give clues as to how influential the message might be.
- USE PROBE QUESTIONS TO ELICIT REASON FOR CHOICES. Sample question: "Would your family or friends probably do _____?" Probe follows: (If either yes or no), "Could you tell me why?"

KEEP TRACK OF THE PURPOSE OF QUESTIONS

As you draft the questions, make a marginal note on the purpose that each question is to serve: i.e., attraction, comprehension, self-efficacy, cultural acceptability, persuasion. These notations help later when compiling the responses. They also serve as a reminder to be sure you've considered all the relevant purposes for the questions. Box 10-1 is an example of a questionnaire showing the purpose of the question on the left side and the questions on the right side. The order of the questions follows the flow of the pamphlet. This is the author's master copy.

CAN YOU USE THE SAME QUESTIONNAIRE FOR SEVERAL INSTRUCTIONS?

Yes and no. Yes for some of the open-ended questions about visuals, comprehension, self-efficacy, and persuasion. No for the specific words, behaviors, information details, artwork, layout, and cultural suitability that relate to a specific instruction.

In summary, questions are derived from the objective and the key points of the instruction that you determine at the beginning of the procedure. For

BOX 10-1

*A completed
questionnaire could look
like this one for the
osteoporosis pamphlet*

FUNCTION	QUESTION
Comprehension	1. Tell me, in your own words, what is this all about? Anything else?
Attraction	2. Let's look at the cover. Would you want to pick it up and read it? (If no, could you tell me why not?)
Comprehension	3. What does the picture of the two women tell you?
Comprehension	4. Turn to inside (p. 1). What's a common name for osteoporosis? How serious is it? Do people die from it?
Comprehension	5. (bottom picture, p. 1) What does this picture tell you?
Self-efficacy	6. Do you think you could do what the picture suggests?
Self-efficacy	7. Here's a list of things some women do (Bone-Robbing Habits). Do you find anything here that you do?
Persuasion	(If yes) Would you change if you knew it might hurt you?
Comprehension	8. How could you find out if you have osteoporosis?
Comprehension	9. (go to next page) What can you do to keep from getting osteoporosis?
Comprehension	10. (Point to food list) What does this list tell you to do?
Comprehension	11. Where could you go to find out if you have osteoporosis?
Acceptability	12. Is there anything in this pamphlet that makes you uncomfortable or is not acceptable for you or your friends?
Persuasion	13. Do you think you might get a test now for osteoporosis?
Persuasion	14. Do you think your family or friends might get a test?

the osteoporosis pamphlet, the four key points determined earlier deal mainly with understanding about osteoporosis. Therefore, most of the questions focus on comprehension. In the poster example (Figure 10-1), recognition of the fruits and vegetables in the visual and eating five of them a day are the key points. If you were testing a procedure to be learned, then a demonstration rather than a questionnaire could be used to see if the patient could carry out the procedure using the set of instructions provided.

The results of testing the nutrition poster and the pamphlet on osteoporosis are given in the Evaluation section later in this chapter. Each interview took about 15 minutes.

A note of caution about self-administered questionnaires: They are much less reliable than interviews. For respondents who do not read well, the responses will have little validity. They tend to skip over items, leaving you with incomplete data. They may go back and change their answers as they get farther into the questionnaire.[9] They often have someone else fill out forms for them, so there is no assurance that *your* respondent actually completed the form. Furthermore, there is less "richness" in the responses because amplifying probe questions are not likely to be asked or responded to.

Train interviewers

For an instruction intended for in-house use at a hospital or clinic, you can conduct the interviews yourself. You can easily interview 10 or more patients in one morning. If you choose to have a larger sample interviewed, you may want to get help. If so, the interviewers will need a little training.

CONTENT OF INTERVIEWER TRAINING

The interviewers need orientation to the material to be tested and the particulars of your plan; you also need to train them in the unique characteristics of learner verification and revision. This is a fact-finding interview, not an instructional session. Therefore, record verbatim answers without trying to paraphrase them.

Training with role-playing could be done in an hour or so, depending on the experience of the interviewers. Some interviewers prefer to work in pairs: one interviews and one records. Additional tips for interviewers are in Appendix D. Appendix D also includes a questionnaire for the interviewers to evaluate their experience.

Plan the sample and select test sites

The nature of the message may appear to dictate the gender of your respondents (i.e., prostate surgery for men and OB/GYN for women). However, the authors suggest including a sample of both men and women for most tests. The influence of the other gender can be a force in carrying out the instruction.

For example, in testing a narrative instruction about two women losing weight, male respondents expressed considerable interest in knowing what kind of food habits were being promoted. They wanted to reinforce and support the efforts of the women.

SIZE OF SAMPLE:

As mentioned earlier in the Overview, learner verification and revision is formative research, so large samples are not needed. You may need to go beyond the 30–50 sample for national distribution and the l0 for local use for the following reasons:

- The length of your material may require a larger sample: Long booklets and long videos increase the likelihood of people missing information, especially near the end. A total of 50 tests is sufficient to pick up what some people may miss.
- The span of cultural diversity desired may require a larger sample: Factors to consider include inner city versus rural; country of origin, especially within the Hispanic culture, because Mexican, Puerto Rican, Central and South American cultures vary markedly. Differences can vary as much between tribal groups (i.e., Native Americans) as between people of different racial backgrounds.

SELECT TEST SITES

Sites may be hospitals (inpatient or outpatient) clinics, health departments, senior centers, adult basic education classes, or other locations where the intended audience is likely to be found. Other locations include central location intercept interviews, theater testing, and gatekeeper reviews. Comparative advantages of these various locations are discussed in recent low literacy and health education program guides.[10,11]

A note of caution: If you delegate testing to subcontractors or to others, make certain the patient samples are drawn from the intended low literacy audiences. For example, community adult literacy programs are appropriate. The authors have had experience with "low literacy" samples taken on college campuses. Do not rely on entry-level unlicensed personnel or clerical staff as substitutes for your intended audience. They are likely to be more familiar with health care terms and jargon.

Step 2: Interview respondents

Tips for interviewers

1. There are no right or wrong answers. This is a fact-finding interview, not an instructional session.
2. People with low literacy skills often lack fluency in vocabulary. Try not to prompt the respondent. Broken sentences with "he" and "she" (unidentified) are common.
3. Gentle refocusing of attention back to the test material is often needed.[12] For example, we had a client tell the story of his brother's leg amputation instead of responding to a direct question about the signs of high blood sugar in a diabetes pamphlet.
4. The introduction of the interview is important. "Would you help me?" at the the end of the introduction sets the stage and creates a mood for cooperation and partnership. The authors have used an introduction like the following:

   "Hello. I'm Ms/Mr. _____ working here at the clinic on some new health instructions. We want them to be attractive, useful, and easy-to-read. I'd appreciate it if you'd read this pamphlet. When you've finished I'd like to ask you some questions to see if we got the important points across. This pamphlet can still be changed, so your opinion can make a difference. There are no right or wrong answers. Would you help me?"

   Most people enjoy having a professional person ask for their opinion and will give time for the interview. Respondents are often quite willing to give advice on how to improve the visuals. The authors have found that clients at clinics, hospitals, senior centers, etc., are willing to be interviewed on a voluntary, nonpaid basis.
5. Test in the same language used in the instruction. For example, don't substitute an English version if the instruction is going to be used in another language. Each language has its own speech patterns, idioms, metaphors, and thought patterns.

An Alternative Method (used by AHEC, Biddeford, Maine)[13]

A combination of individual and group testing methods has also proven effective in assessing short instructions such as single-sheet, onefold pamphlets. The following example illustrates this dual testing approach and how to do it using the literacy, health, and education resources within the community. Salient characteristics of this approach are:

1. Individual assessment by a written checklist, customized for the pamphlet
2. Group interview to obtain additional responses about comprehension, self-efficacy, persuasion, and to obtain suggestions to improve the material (standardized questionnaire for group interview)
3. The use of adult basic education or other specific group resources for leaders and for target audience

Method: a two-part process:

1. Individual assessment (via a checklist)
2. Group interviews

Who conducts it: collaborative learner verification and revision testing with adult basic education and health care professionals

Small group setting: 8–10 adults

Two leaders: one from the health field; one from adult basic literacy field

Time: 1–2 hours total (including both Parts 1 and 2)

Target audience: adult basic education students (method has also been used with Women Infant Children Program, Head Start, drug counseling units, and select patient groups)

Materials needed

FOR INDIVIDUAL ASSESSMENT FOR EACH RESPONDENT:

1. Draft copy of new pamphlet (collected later along with completed checklist)
2. Customized checklist designed to determine how well the respondent understands the three or four key points of the pamphlet (sample: Fig. 10-6. Author of pamphlet develops checklist in collaboration with literacy/ health professionals.)
3. Pencils

FOR GROUP INTERVIEWS BY LEADERS

1. Draft copies of new pamphlet
2. Standardized discussion guide

PART 1: Individual responses with written checklist:

• All respondents in the group are asked to read the draft pamphlet by themselves.

- Upon completion of the reading, a checklist is given to each person to complete without referring to the pamphlet.
- To test their remembering the information, the respondents check boxes, circles, or underline answers. Language on the checklist is the same as in the pamphlet. This is based on the assumption that if they could read the words in the booklet, they could also read the checklist. Leaders collect unsigned checklists.

Figure 10-6 is a partial copy of a checklist used for a pamphlet, "Good News for Older Smokers."

FIGURE 10-6

The checklist keeps attention focused on what the pamphlet says. (*Source: Over 60 Health Center Smoking Cessation Program, 1860 Alcatraz, Berkeley, CA 94703*)

GOOD NEWS FOR OLDER SMOKERS

After you have read the booklet, please put it aside and answer these questions. We want to see if the booklet was clearly written. This is not a test of you—it is a test of the booklet.

Please put a check in each box that tells you something that you read in the booklet.

If you stop smoking, you will:
- ☐ Cut down on the risk of stroke or heart attack.
- ☐ Cut down on colds.
- ☐ Save money.
- ☐ Feel better about yourself.
- ☐ Not gain weight.
- ☐ Smell better.

People smoke more:
- ☐ The older they get.
- ☐ When they do things like driving, watching TV or telephoning.
- ☐ When they are bored, lonely or angry.
- ☐ When they are away from home.

Put a check on the things the booklet suggested you do instead of smoking:
- ☐ Close your eyes and take ten deep breaths.
- ☐ Listen to music and sing along or dance.
- ☐ Chew gum.
- ☐ Brush your teeth.
- ☐ Bake a cake or pie.
- ☐ Call someone on the phone.
- ☐ Eat a piece of fruit.
- ☐ Go fishing
- ☐ Drink a glass of water.
- ☐ Take a walk.

PART 2: Group interviews using a standardized guide such as the following:

Questions for Group Review

These questions are discussion starters. You may need to probe for more specific information, depending on the answers to these kinds of general questions. Have a colleague record responses and/or use a tape recorder.

1. What are some words you would use to describe this pamphlet?
2. Is there any new information in this pamphlet? If so, what?
3. Is the information doable? That is, could you use the ideas in your own life? If not, what doesn't make sense or doesn't seem useful?
4. Would you be willing to try the ideas? Why or why not?
5. Are any words hard for you? Which ones?
6. How do the pictures help get the message across?
7. Is the print big enough? Too big?
8. Can you think of ways this pamphlet could be improved?

Summary of Parts 1 and 2: The objectives of the material and the key points must be identified regardless of what interviewing method you use. It is also important to try to identify the problem words, artwork, and layout for each instruction.

The choice is in the selection of the interviewing method. Should you use a personal interview one-on-one method? The advantages of one-on-one are:

1. You can carry it out with a few patients or clients in an office, in a clinic, on the street, or wherever the setting permits.
2. It offers privacy and confidentiality for the respondent.
3. It offers opportunity for in-depth respondent replies and for probe questions, and provides quantitative data on the responses.
4. There is great flexibility for timing when interviews are to be conducted.
5. It is suitable for assessing material of any length, in any medium.

Should you use the interview/group discussion method? The advantages are:

1. Responses from the group can trigger additional information that may clarify or amplify points.
2. It offers group reaction and/or support for thoughts and ideas.
3. The group can be constructed to meet certain specifications, i.e., randomized or selected.
4. Evaluation and assessment of changes for revision may benefit from the group leader's interpretation.

Whatever method or combination of methods you choose, by all means verify the suitability of the material with your audience.

Step 3: Evaluate responses and revise

Tabulating responses

For small samples: A simple tabular form may be sufficient. Displaying the responses to each question in tabular form is helpful because you can quickly spot problems with the material. A series of partially correct or wrong responses to a question often becomes evident with as few as 4 or 5 responses tabulated.

For large samples: See Appendix D, Figure D-1: sample computer spreadsheet.

Evaluating responses

As Wright points out, not only is there no magical figure that can be pinned on a text as some sort of seal of approval, but it is clearly meaningless to look at average figures for the total text, such as a 15-percent error rate. There are very different redesign implications depending on whether the problems occur scattered throughout the material, whether they are localized, and the level of confidence you need in having people understand the message.[14] For example, missing a descriptive passage is not as significant as missing the dosage for a medication.

The tabulated data allow you to evaluate the responses in terms of each question, as well as in terms of each respondent. You can evaluate each question by counting the numbers of responses that were correct, partly correct, and wrong. This simple evaluation is often quite revealing.

When you evaluate by respondent, you may find that some respondents give wrong responses to most of the questions. What is it about these respondents that may be the cause of their not getting it? Both cuts of the data can be useful. Evaluations can also be made in terms of the function of the question, i.e., comprehension, acceptability, etc.

These different cuts of the data can uncover unsuspected problems. For example, the responses may show that most people understand the message and find it culturally acceptable. However, a self-efficacy question may show that the respondents don't believe they could do what the instruction asks of them. This finding could lead to a suggestion to retain the existing content, but to repackage it into a number of small, easy-to-do steps. Or perhaps it may point to the need to add supporting testimonials of others who adopted the behaviors called for in the instruction.

Cross-correlations between the respondents' demographics and the questions with incorrect responses can also be revealing. For example, one may find that nearly all of the incorrect responses to a question were made by respondents over 60 years of age. Such a finding may lead to an assessment of the readability of that part of the text in the instructional material because, as noted in Chapter 1, people over age 60 have a much higher incidence of functional illiteracy. Perhaps they couldn't read that part of the material!

Revising the instruction

How should you decide from the learner verification and revision responses whether or not changes are really needed? How many wrong answers warrant the decision to change?—a step that could have significant cost impact if the instruction is in final form ready for production. Make the decision based on the following criteria:

1. The importance of the wrong responses in terms of the purpose and key points previously identified for the material.
2. The number of respondents who got it wrong.
3. The cultural acceptance and self-efficacy responses: if either of these two factors had a high number of wrong or negative responses, the material should be revised.

It would be convenient to have threshold numbers to revise or not revise for the criteria above, but the threshold depends on the importance of the information for the use of each material. For example, where the information deals with safety of life there should be a zero or near zero tolerance for incorrect responses.

Even if only 5 percent of respondents replied incorrectly to a comprehension question on a key point, a revision or a reassessment should be made. On the other hand, if the material assessed is intended to serve a multi-cultural population, some cultural mismatch is to be expected and a higher tolerance (percentage) of unfavorable responses may be acceptable (perhaps 10 percent) without making any change.

To sum up the evaluation: classify passages of the text in terms of the tolerance of misunderstanding that will be accepted. If the differences are with nice-to-know but not critical information, such as statistics, then it may not be cost-effective to make expensive revisions. On the other hand, if there is misunderstanding of the key points of the instruction, extensive revision may be needed.

Although the immediate results of evaluation are diagnostic for that specific instruction, there is a long-term advantage to keeping track of these problems so that you can avoid them in the future. These problems can range from graphics to vocabulary and it is not easy to generalize after assessing only one instruction. However, over time after learner verification and revision assessment of several materials, patterns of problems may become evident and these may be dealt with more systematically for future materials.

Examples of results from learner verification and revision testing

Three examples provide a range of data to show what you might expect from testing typical health instructions.

Example 1: Box 10-2 is from a pamphlet urging a change of diet to reduce cancer risks by eating cruciferous vegetables. "Cruciferous" was reworded to "in the cabbage family." However, many people still had no idea what that meant. They couldn't respond to this question.

BOX 10-2

*Sample of test check list
on nutrition pamphlet.
(Source: The Good Life,
American Cancer
Society, 1599 Clifton Rd.
NE Atlanta, GA 30329)*

CIRCLE ALL THE FOODS IN THE CABBAGE FAMILY:		
cauliflower	brussel sprouts	turnip greens
carrots	celery sticks	chic peas
lettuce	kale	cole slaw

Recommendations for revision: The pamphlet needs to have visuals and greater detail of the size, shape, and texture of vegetables to help people recognize "the cabbage family."

Example 2: Figure 10-1, the poster, "Your doctor wants you to eat five fruits and vegetables a day." Findings are organized according to the key points tested:

1. Your doctor wants you to eat five fruits and vegetables every day.
2. Identify fruits and vegetables pictured.
3. Fruits and vegetables taste great; they cost is less in season.

Findings: The "five-a-day" was well understood. However, the credibility of the message failed. Doctors are perceived as persuading people to change behavior for health reasons, not for taste and cost. It doesn't make sense. Only 51 percent thought that it was a persuasive message. The poster is perceived more as a grocery ad than as advice from doctors.

"Identify the fruits and vegetables pictured": A large number, 88 percent, did not recognize romaine lettuce. Some thought it was a type of lettuce, but they "ate iceberg." Others thought it was bok choy, broccoli, or kale. Some confused asparagus with celery, but the majority who recognized asparagus were emphatic in saying they would not eat it.

Recommendations for revision: Some major revisions are indicated by the confusion with the key points:

1. Change the subtitle about taste and cost to conform with expectations about doctors' advice, i.e., "Vegetables cut your risk of cancer."
2. Change romaine lettuce to a more familiar vegetable.
3. Change asparagus to one that is better liked.
4. Label each vegetable and fruit

Example 3: Figures 10-2 through 10-5, the pamphlet, "Osteoporosis and You." Findings are organized according to the key points tested:

1. Understanding what osteoporosis is
2. Identifying risk factors you can change
3. Understanding what to do to prevent osteoporosis
4. Knowing how to detect it

Findings: The concept of osteoporosis and risk factors are only partially understood. The following range of responses shows some confusion and an association with *parts* of the explanation given in the pamphlet: "It's about bone disease"; "a disease of the joints"; "I didn't understand it"; "foods you *should* eat"; "people with broken hips can die"; "osteoporosis, bones break easily."

The term "hunchback" is a little better understood: "thin bones or something"; "a bone disease;" "broken bones"; "arthritis;" "it's hunch back."

People understood the preventive behaviors better than the concept of bone thinning and loss of calcium. Examples of their responses are: "take calcium"; "change diet"; "exercise"; "eating habits, exercise"; "eat foods high in calcium."

People understood how osteoporosis could be detected. All understood that you went to a doctor for a test. Forty percent knew the test procedure was either scan or x-ray and another 40 percent knew you went to Queens Hospital.

Recommendations for revision: Responses indicate a need for redesign and revision changes:

1. Shift the concept to "hunch back." Use the Health Belief Model to reorganize the sequence of information. Emphasize "you." Either drop or explain "bone thinning and robbing" with examples.
2. Write "hunch back" as a caption and emphasize with an arrow.
3. One picture of the hunchback on the cover makes the message clear.
4. "Chunk" the long lists of preventive actions to understand easier.
5. On the diet list, rank the high-calcium-content foods first.

Advice: For already published material that will not likely be revised soon, consider writing an insert sheet that clarifies or simplifies the information. It can also provide additional advice.

Terminating the revision process

Deciding when to terminate the revision process is really an arbitrary decision. It is well to keep in mind that several drafts are likely to be tested before arriving at a satisfactory instruction. A rule of thumb is to test major redesign features after each draft. Small wording changes may not be necessary to retest.

Often several people or a committee are involved in the design and/or approval process for materials. In these circumstances, let the learner verification and revision data serve as your verification. Many health care professionals do not understand the kind of changes necessary for low literacy patients. So when you present your draft along with the results of your testing, the information speaks for itself.

Learner Verification and Revision for Questionnaires, Audiotapes, Videotapes, and Demonstrations

Questionnaires

Questionnaires are increasingly used for behavioral research in health care for minorities as well as for health promotion programs in smoking cessation, cholesterol control, etc.

We recommend two steps in verification of questionnaires:[15]

1. Test the questionnaire with a small sample of the intended audience to verify that they understand the questions the way you intend:

   (a) Not every question is tested, but key questions need to be identified.

   (b) Questions like these help to clarify the intent of the question:
   — What did the question mean to you?
   — (when person hesitates) What made it hard for you to answer?
   — What further ideas do you have that were not brought out by the question?
   — How would you ask the question?
   — How do you feel about questions that you answered "I don't know"?

2. Obtain feedback from interviewers: the interviewer also provides valuable information. Some of these questions could help improve your planning as well as programming:

   — What problems did you have in locating respondents and in interviewing?

   — What points seemed to cause embarrassment or resistance?

   — Where did you have trouble maintaining rapport?

   — Were the respondents bored or impatient?

   — What questions brought forth interest in further information?

   — Did you have enough space for recording answers?

Audiotapes

Planning: Use the same planning steps described earlier in this chapter: i.e., identifying the key points, writing the questions. Unique to audiotape testing are the following elements:

- Is the pacing of the story or the information about right? "Did you slowly get bored?" "Was it easy to follow the tape?" Did people talk too slow, too fast, or about right?"
- Is the story culturally suitable? "Did the people sound like people from around here?" In testing a tape produced in another language, for example,

Spanish, you want to know if the accent, vocabulary, and examples used in the tape are suitable for your audience.[16]
- Is the audio reproduction of good quality? "Could you hear them okay?"
- If sound effects were used, "Could you tell what the sound meant when . . . ?"
- If music was used, "Is this the kind of music you like?"

Interviewing: Ask the client to listen to the tape and essentially use the same introduction as you would for text, except the client listens to the tape and you ask questions afterward. A comment from one patient was, "When I read, I just go on and on and I don't know what I've read. But with a tape, I listen right along with people and it's easier."

Video

Planning: Use the same planning steps described in this chapter, i.e., clearly state objectives, identify the key points, and write the questions. For video, group interviews are probably more efficient than individual interviews. Unique features of testing video are:

- In the draft stage, use a set of story boards to test the key points. The client looks at the story board while you read the script or have a tape recorder play the sound for you. How well do the video and audio synchronize for the learner? Does the video match the audio? Does it move too fast or too slowly?

FOR VIDEOS ON THE MARKET:

- Preview a video two or three times to be sure you have identified all the key points.
- Consider asking questions about any text shown. Sometimes the text is shown for only a few seconds. Did the text stay on the screen long enough for you to get it?
- Cultural appropriateness is indicated by dress, appearance, speech, background setting, and mannerisms. Do these people look like your friends or family?

Interviewing: Introduce the video by describing what it is about, who the characters are, how long it is, and any special details that you want respondents to look for, i.e., steps in a procedure and use of color. Show the video and then ask the questions as you would in a group discussion.

Demonstrations

Planning: The objective of the demonstration and the key points needed for comprehension need to be clearly identified ahead of time.

Demonstrating: Introduce the subject, tell what you are going to do, and tell the person/group that you are going to ask each of them to do the procedure immediately after you finish.

Individual demonstration: Prepare the same setup the way you had it before you started. Keep your copy of the procedure with you. Ask the person to go ahead and carry out the procedure the way you did it. Make note of where the person bogs down and has trouble remembering what to do next. The hesitations and slowing down tell you these are trouble spots. If possible, do not interrupt until the person is through.

Demonstration for a group: If the subject is suitable, have the group divide into pairs and demonstrate to each other. Again, make note of where people seem uncertain or hesitate to take the next step. Conduct a discussion afterward on what they found easy, where they experienced trouble, and what additional help they feel they need.

References

1. This chapter updates Chapter 9, Pretesting, in the 1985 edition of this book.
2. Veermeeersch JA and Swenerton H (1980): Interpretations of nutrition claims in food and advertisements by low-income consumers. J. Nutrition Education 12(1):19–25 as contained in Rudd, et al. (January–Februaty 1993): Developing written nutrition information for adults with low literacy skills. J. Nutrition Education 15(1): 11–16.
3. Samora J, et al. (1961): Medical vocabulary knowledge among hospital patients. J Health and Human Behavior 2:83–92.
4. Larrabee P (1977): Masters thesis, Patients' understanding of vocabulary terms used in initial health assessments, University of Rochester, School of Nursing, Rochester, NY. Available on microfilm from University Microfilms International, Ann Arbor, Michigan, 48106, and London, England.
5. Selman S (1994): Personal communication.
6. Rudd J, et al. (January–February 1993): Developing written nutrition information for adults with low literacy skills. J Nutrition Education 25(l):11–16.
7. Hosey GM, et al. (1991): Designing and evaluating diabetes education material for American Indians. Diabetes Educator 16(5):407–414.
8. Stanton M (1989): Personal communication.
9. Bertrand JT (1978): Communications Pretesting, Media Monograph 6, Communication Laboratory, Community and Family Study Center, University of Chicago, 1411 E. 60th St., Chicago, IL 60637.
10. Beyond the Brochure: Alternative Approaches to Effective Health Communication (1994): AMC Cancer Research Center, Denver, CO, and the Centers for Disease Control and Prevention, Atlanta, GA.
11. Making Health Communication Programs Work: A Planner's Guide (April 1992): USHHS, Public Health Service, Office of Cancer Communication, NCI, NIH Publication No. 92-1493.
12. Doak C, Doak L, Root J (1985): Teaching Patients with Low Literacy Skills. Philadelphia: Lippincott. See Chapter 1, The problem, pp. 7–8.
13. AHEC Office, University of New England, Biddeford, ME. Supported by AHEC and The Bingham Foundation, 1990–1993.
14. Wright P (1985): The Technology of Text, DH Jonassen (ed), Vol. 2. Englewood Cliffs, NJ: Educational Technology Publications. See Chapter 18, Is evaluation a myth? Assessing text assessment procedures.
15. Selltiz J, et al. (1966): Research Methods in Social Relations. Holt, Rhinehart and Winston New York, NY, p. 551.
16. The authors tested a dialogue tape recorded in Spanish with one speaker from Columbia, South America, and the other from Puerto Rico. The largely Puerto Rican audience commented immediately that the Columbian "doesn't talk like us." The different accent created dissonance and the message needed to be retaped with two Puerto Ricans.

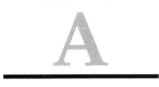

Appendix

A

Literacy Data and Measures

Defining Literacy/Illiteracy

During the 1800s, people were deemed literate if they could write their own names. Today, people need much higher literacy skills to understand their health-care instructions and to function in society.

Until a few years ago, literacy skills were universally measured in terms of **grade level**—the average reading skill level achieved at each year of schooling in the American school system. Readability difficulty of text was also rated by school grade level. This system is in wide use today.

More recently, literacy skills (as well as the literacy demand of materials) are sometimes defined in terms of **competency level** via measures of task difficulty. Descriptions of both the grade level and competency measures follow.

Grade-level measures of literacy

There is no universally accepted definition of literacy or illiteracy. Cook (1977) cites the U.S. Army's definition of literacy in terms of reading skills at a minimum grade level—the 5th grade.[1] This level was commensurate with the reading demands of the simplest of the Army's training manuals. Those who had reading/writing skills at or above 5th grade could read the manuals and were literate; those reading below this level were termed functionally illiterate. This definition is widely shared today, although the word *illiterate* is falling into disuse.

The use of grade levels for reading skills by the Army not only reflects the nation's school systems, but also the scale used by the most widely used reading assessment instrument in the health community: the Wide Range Achievement Test (WRAT).[2] Grade-level measurements have advantages and disadvantages.

A significant advantage is that grade level is widely understood in the United States as a measuring scale for literacy skills. A further advantage is that, for materials, readability formulas also report reading difficulty in terms of grade level. By measuring reading skills of people and the readability of materials on the same scale, we can easily see if the materials are at a suitable level.

A disadvantage is that most reading skill instruments measure a person's skills at reading text only, but do not measure skills in visual reading, including charts, graphs, and problem solving. Another disadvantage is that adults often develop more advanced skills to read a subject of special interest to them, but such skills would not be detected by the testing instruments.

Competency measures of literacy

Since the mid-1970s, a competency-based scale for both people's reading skills and the difficulty of written materials has been developed and used in the National Adult Literacy Surveys (NALS). A scale of zero (lowest/easiest) to 500 (highest/most difficult) is used for rating both people and the text and numeracy materials. These scores are grouped into five levels:

Level 1	0 to 225	(lowest/simplest)
Level 2	226 to 275	
Level 3	276 to 325	
Level 4	326 to 375	
Level 5	376 to 500	(highest/most complex)

An advantage of the zero to 500 rating scale is that it has broader applications than the grade-level scale. It applies to tasks included in prose, document, and numeracy materials. The reading formulas mentioned earlier apply to text only and without regard to the difficulty of tasks, such as numeracy or graphic tasks, which may be necessary to use the materials.

A major disadvantage of the zero to 500 scale is that its meaning and interpretation are largely unknown to health-care professionals. Health-care materials may contain a number of topics and tasks and it would be difficult to arrive at a single collective rating using the zero to 500 scale. The authors recognize both scales, but in the interest of making this book of immediate use to health-care professionals, the grade-level scale is used predominantly.

Competency scales pose a dilemma for health-care practitioners who want to measure the literacy levels of materials they develop or use on the zero to 500 scale. If they use the extensive NALS survey data about literacy competency, how can they use the same scale to measure the competency demand of their health instructions? There is no convenient formula to use.

The NALS uses three criteria to establish a rating on the scale:

1. The structure of the material (i.e., narrative, chart, graph)
2. The content and/or context
3. The nature of the task that must be done

Since the NALS is a research-based project in literacy, it has not provided a "formula" to apply the three criteria to health-care materials. Furthermore, the NALS competency questions are usually quite brief—at most half a page—and are of the same structure throughout. In contrast, health-care instructions may be several pages long and often consist of several kinds of structure (narrative, tables, graphs, illustrations, etc.)

One way to apply the NALS criteria to health-care materials may be to partition the health instruction and analyze parts of like structure. That is, obtain a NALS score for each part. This seems rather tedious, and we have requested a more suitable approach from the NALS authors.

Magnitude of the Literacy Problem

National literacy surveys conducted since the 1970s have consistently shown that between 16 and 20 percent of adult Americans are functionally illiterate.[3] Profiles of national literacy in terms of both grade levels and competency levels are shown in Figure 1-1 in Chapter 1. The national data in competency terms for prose, document, and quantitative literacy are shown in Figure A-1.

FIGURE A-1

Literacy levels of the total U.S. population. (*Source: National Adult Literacy Survey, U.S. Department of Education, 1993*)

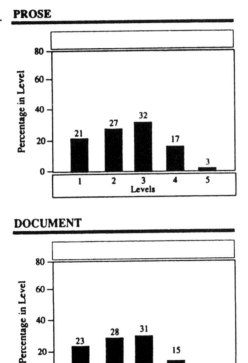

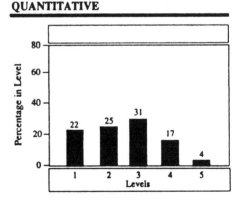

The results show 21 to 23 percent in level one. These people, on average, will understand little from most current health instructions.

When we combine the 21 percent at level 1 with the additional 27 percent of marginal readers at level 2, we see that literacy problems are experienced by nearly half of the U.S. population. This population group will either not understand or will have difficulty with most written health care instructions.

Literacy surveys have also been conducted by a number of states including Oregon, Mississippi, Florida, and Hawaii. Some state surveys use the same questions and rating scales as the NALS.[4]

Age and ethnic considerations

Literacy skills vary by age and by ethnic group. Older people, those 65 and over, have much lower literacy skills. Forlizi (1989) points out that functional illiteracy among this group is about 35 percent—about double that of the population as a whole. NALS data show that document literacy skills of the 65 and older group drop to level 1 compared to level 3 for the 25 to 39 age group.

Literacy skills of ethnic groups are lower than that of the U.S. population as a whole. Their lower performance stems from the influence of a number of variables, including years of schooling. Functional illiteracy is more prevalent among ethnic groups, and for one Southeast Asian group, it reaches a level above 50 percent.[5] The NALS report shows that literacy skills of American ethnic groups average one level lower than the general population.

What does this mean to you as a health-care provider? Clearly, you may have to use instructions at lower literacy levels for older people, for ethnic groups, and indeed, for a great part of the U.S. population. Since these groups have such sizable numbers of people with low reading skills, consider including alternative media such as simple visuals, demonstrations, verbal or audio-taped instructions instead of text.

Literacy skills of patients has an impact on costs for their health care. Weiss (1992) points out that those with the lowest levels of literacy skills are likely to incur health-care costs that are many times higher than people with even marginal literacy skills.[6]

References

1. Cook DW (1977): Adult Literacy Education in the United States. International Reading Association, p. 68. Newark, DE.
2. The Wide Range Achievement Test (WRAT 3) (1993): Newark, DE: Jastak Inc.
3. Forlizi LA (1989): Adult literacy in the United States today. Report from the Institute for the Study of Adult Literacy. University Park, PA: Penn State University.
4. Oregon Progress Board (May 1991): The Oregon Literacy Survey. Salem, OR: Economic Development Department.
5. Dehn RW, Schneider DM (November 1989): Patient Literacy in a Family Practice Clinic. Presentation at American Academy of Family Physicians, Orlando, FL.
6. Weiss BD, et al. (May–June 1992): Health status of illiterate adults: relation between literacy and health status among persons with low literacy skills. Journal of American Board of Family Practice 5(3):257–264.

REALM

RAPID ESTIMATE OF ADULT LITERACY IN MEDICINE
(REALM)©

Terry Davis, PhD • Michael Crouch, MD • Sandy Long, PhD

Patient Name/
Subject # _____ Date of Birth _____

Reading
Level _____

Grade
Completed _____

Date _____ Clinic _____ Examiner _____

List 1		List 2		List 3	
fat	_____	fatigue	_____	allergic	_____
flu	_____	pelvic	_____	menstrual	_____
pill	_____	jaundice	_____	testicle	_____
dose	_____	infection	_____	colitis	_____
eye	_____	exercise	_____	emergency	_____
stress	_____	behavior	_____	medication	_____
smear	_____	prescription	_____	occupation	_____
nerves	_____	notify	_____	sexually	_____
germs	_____	gallbladder	_____	alcoholism	_____
meals	_____	calories	_____	irritation	_____
disease	_____	depression	_____	constipation	_____
cancer	_____	miscarriage	_____	gonorrhea	_____
caffeine	_____	pregnancy	_____	inflammatory	_____
attack	_____	arthritis	_____	diabetes	_____
kidney	_____	nutrition	_____	hepatitis	_____
hormones	_____	menopause	_____	antibiotics	_____
herpes	_____	appendix	_____	diagnosis	_____
seizure	_____	abnormal	_____	potassium	_____
bowel	_____	syphilis	_____	anemia	_____
asthma	_____	hemorrhoids	_____	obesity	_____
rectal	_____	nausea	_____	osteoporosis	_____
incest	_____	directed	_____	impetigo	_____

SCORE
List 1 _____
List 2 _____
List 3 _____
Raw Score _____

RAPID ESTIMATE OF ADULT LITERACY IN MEDICINE

The Rapid Estimate of Adult Literacy in Medicine (REALM) is a screening instrument to assess an adult patient's ability to read common medical words and lay terms for body parts and illnesses. It is designed to assist medical professionals in estimating a patient's literacy level so that the appropriate level of patient education materials or oral instructions may be used. The test takes 2 to 3 minutes to administer and score. The REALM has been correlated with other standardized tests.

Correlation of REALM with SORT, PIAT-R, and WRAT-R			
	PIAT-R Recognition	SORT	WRAT-R
Correlation Coefficient	.97	.96	.88
P Value	p<.0001	p<.0001	p<.0001

Reliability Studies	
Test-Retest	Inter-Rater
(n = 100)	(n = 20)
.99	.99

DIRECTIONS:

1. Give the patient a laminated copy of the REALM and score answers on an unlaminated copy that is attached to a clipboard. Hold the clipboard at an angle so that the patient is not distracted by your scoring procedure. Say:

   "I want to hear you read as many words as you can from this list. Begin with the first word on List 1 and read aloud. When you come to a word you cannot read, do the best you can or say "blank" and go on to the next word."

2. If the patient takes more than five seconds on a word, say "blank" and point to the next word, if necessary, to move the patient along. If the patient begins to miss every word, have him/her pronounce only known words.

3. Count as an error any word not attempted or mispronounced. Score by marking a plus (+) after each correct word, a check (√) after each mispronounced word, and a minus (-) after words not attempted. Count as correct any self-corrected word.

4. Count the number of correct words for each list and record the numbers in the "SCORE" box. Total the numbers and match the total score with its grade equivalent in the table below.

| | **GRADE EQUIVALENT** |
Raw Score	Grade Range
0-18	**3rd Grade and Below** Will not be able to read most low literacy materials; will need repeated oral instructions, materials composed primarily of illustrations, or audio or video tapes.
19-44	**4th to 6th Grade** Will need low literacy materials; may not be able to read prescription labels.
45-60	**7th to 8th Grade** Will struggle with most patient education materials; will not be offended by low literacy materials.
61-66	**High School** Will be able to read most patient education materials.

Used with permission of Terry Davis, Louisiana State University.

Tips for Low-Cost Production

You have done the development work on a pamphlet, form, or instruction sheet, you have checked with other professionals, and you are ready to get the views of your target audience. You will need a copy of your materials that looks as good as you can make it. The suggestions that follow will help you through the production stage of the work, even if you have only the most modest copying and word-processing equipment.

Layout

The layout *is* important. The blocks of text and illustrations on a page should be comfortable—neither too widely spaced nor too close together. Lists spread out down the page may be far more attractive (and easier to read) if items are gathered together in the center of the page with a relevant illustration or two to warm things up. One way to check on page organization is to squint your eyes so the print is blurred and only the blocks of print and white spaces are apparent. If it looks awkward or spotty when viewed this way, it probably is awkward and spotty. In general, it's well to leave slightly more space in the margin at the bottom than at the top. Side margins are equal to or slightly less than top margins.

If you have desktop publishing equipment, you can produce the whole page on the computer at one time regardless of page shape. Your computer may not do that, and you may have to arrange blocks of print or illustrations physically to get a page layout to your liking. A procedure to do this is outlined on the following pages.

Cutting out blocks of text and graphics:

- Cut out blocks of the text and the illustrations you will use, being careful to cut them with square corners.
- Place them on a paper of finished size.
- Put a second sheet of *lined* paper underneath to serve as guidelines to keep

your blocks horizontal. (You may have to make the lines darker so they will show through.) An alternative is to use a drafting table, a T-square, and a triangle, which will speed up your work.

• Put masking tape on the corners of these two sheets to hold them on the desk.

Now you are ready to move your blocks of print and illustrations around on the page.

Preliminary layout

When you are satisfied with the placement of each block of copy:

1. Put a small piece of masking tape (not transparent tape) on one corner of each block to hold it in place.
2. Carefully line up the lettering and margins for each block using the see-through lines.
3. Fasten each block firmly with another piece of masking tape on the diagonal corner. The result might look like Figure C-1.
4. Now, put a small mark on the other diagonal corners (or along each edge) with a *light blue* pencil, as light blue will not show on a photocopy (Figure C-2).
5. One at a time, remove each block of copy. Cover the back with rubber cement, being sure to put cement on the edges. For most applications, use adhesive only on the back surface of the block to be attached, not on the page.

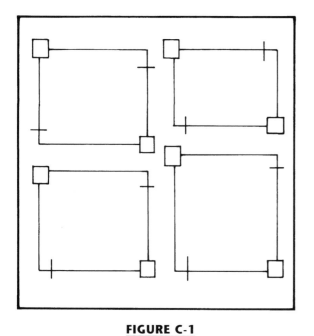

FIGURE C-1

Step 3 in preliminary layout of a page.

FIGURE C-2

Step 4 in page layout.

6. Replace the copy on the page, using the blue lines to guide you. Some repositioning is possible before firmly pressing the block onto the page.
7. Use the back of a spoon to press the edges and corners of the copy tightly against the page.
8. Then, gently use a soft eraser to remove any rubber cement still on the surface. Having glued only one surface, it's still possible to lift a block and try again if you do this shortly after application.

For most applications, use rubber cement adhesive only on the surface to be attached. Place gently. This can be moved slightly, or peeled off. If you want a *permanent* bond, put adhesive on both the back of the block and on the page (only inside the blue lines). Let both surfaces dry until there is no shine to the adhesive. Carefully put the two surfaces together and press firmly. It will be hard to shift this, once bonding has occurred.

When you buy rubber cement in stationery or hardware stores, get the thinner as well. Store your desk bottle upside-down (to exclude air) and thin as needed.

If there is to be a fold in the completed piece, a very small line or dot where the fold is intended will help you in that operation.

Tips on the Copy Machine

What you have been making is called a *mechanical* in printer parlance. Now you are ready to make a master copy. You will probably be using a standard copy machine. Make an initial copy to check placement of your copy on the machine. You may find a shadow line around the edges of the blocks of copy you glued. Push the "Lighter" button on the copy machine. This should remove the shadow lines. If some still remain, you may have to "Lighten" further or use your bottle of white correcting fluid to cover the troubling edges. (The "Lighter" trick also works if you are printing a copy from material on colored paper. By making the copy lighter, the dark background may disappear.)

When you get a copy with good print contrast and no extraneous marks, print two or three copies on laser paper. This high-quality paper is available wherever copy machine supplies are sold. It is super-white and will provide the best possible contrast for the master copies. Write "Master!" on the back (or with your blue pencil on the front) and *always use the master to make copies*. Giving people material to read with broken or faded letters caused by generations of copies is unprofessional. File the mechanical and two extra masters where they will always be available—and never give them away.

You can reach this stage of production before you test your pamphlet with members of your target audience. You may well do all this again when you have adopted suggestions from audience testing. But it takes longer to explain it than to do it. Once you have worked your way through the steps that produce a good mechanical and master, you'll find it's more fun than drudgery.

Obtaining a STAT or PMT

After all the reviewers have had their say, you will make a final mechanical with the corrections you wish to include. If copies are to be produced in your own agency, that may be as far as you need to go. If you wish to go one step further, you can take your mechanical to a graphic arts facility and get a PMT (photo-mechanical transfer) or a stat (short for photostat), which will provide you with the best possible copy from which to make subsequent masters or copies. Stats cost relatively little ($5 to $10) and assure top-quality reproduction. Stats can be damaged by sunlight and should be stored in a filing cabinet.

Graphic Artists and Illustrators

If your budget allows, you can hire a graphic artist and/or an illustrator to do a professional job of illustrating, layout, and design. The graphics designer will work with you on typeface (font), spacing, choice of paper, certain kinds of graphics, such as boxes and picture overlays. The graphics designer works on the overall look you are trying to achieve. The designer may also direct you to an illustrator and may supervise that person if you request it. It usually takes about three months to produce a piece when other professionals are involved. Of course, all this costs money. Be sure you are very clear about *who* does *what*, within what *time schedules*, what happens if you don't agree, and who has final say on process and product. That should all be in writing so there will be no surprises. If you intend to hire professionals, look over their other work (a portfolio) and don't be afraid to ask questions. Two or three bids on a project should give you the information you need to choose wisely.

How or Where Do I Get Illustrations?

There are three major sources for getting illustrations:

1. You may want to employ a professional illustrator. The illustrator will give you several sketches to carry out the ideas you have indicated.
2. If you are on a tight budget, you may have to finish the project yourself. You may be able to find just the illustrations you want in clip art books or a computer graphics program. You can usually buy clip art wherever arts and crafts supplies are sold. If some of the clip art drawings are too shaded (simple line drawings are best) or contain too many distracting details, try correction fluid or cut off the nonessential details.
3. Perhaps you know someone who can produce some drawings for you. It's worth asking at art schools and colleges.

Agreements When Working with Production Professionals

As you work out agreements for the services of people you may hire, specify exactly:

- What is to be done by each one
- Ownership of the materials produced
- Time allowed, with deadlines (if needed)
- Costs of services including revisions

Again, if there's anything you don't understand, don't be afraid to ask questions. If the pamphlet is to be printed, get an estimate of the costs involved.

Printing costs will vary according to:

1. Printing process: offset, copy machine, typeset, etc.
2. Number of copies: cost per copy goes down as quantity goes up.
3. Quality of stock: glossy and heavy equals nice but expensive.
4. Number of colors: each color is a press run.
5. Size of item: standard stock is less expensive.
6. Other operations: folding, stapling, spiralbound, etc.

If the quote you get exceeds your budget, ask your printer's help in trimming the cost by modifying choices in the list above.

Summary

Good presentation is important. You can produce material that looks professional even if it is not "slick." Don't be satisfied with out-of-date, inappropriate, or badly reproduced handouts. Materials with a professional appearance receive greater respect and credibility.

Appendix

D

Learner Verification and Revision

Tips on Interviewing

Q. *What should I do while the person is reading the material?*

A. Have some notes or other reading material with you so that you can be busy looking at something, not looking directly at the person. Some interviewers have found that giving attention to the children (if present) helps.

During the interview

Q. *What's the most important thing to keep in mind while interviewing?*

A. To record exactly what the person says without any interpretation. Broken phrases or slang expressions are important cues for us to learn about language that may communicate more effectively.

Q. *Suppose the person starts asking me questions about what the piece is actually saying. How should I handle these questions?*

A. First of all, jot down his or her questions because these may be important cues for us that the point being made is not clear.

Next, acknowledge the question by saying something like, "I'm glad you asked that question. I'll be glad to talk about that as soon as we finish here. Right now, I'd like to go on to . . .

If you break the train of thought of the interview at this point and digress by giving an explanation, then the whole focus shifts away from the material being tested. It could become a teaching session rather than a learner verification test. You can answer any questions *after* the interview is completed.

Q. *Do I have to ask the questions as written on the questionnaire?*

A. Yes. Consistency is necessary among all the different interviews. Please ask the questions the way they're phrased, and in the sequence they are given. Don't skip around.

Q. *What if I don't understand the answer given to a question I asked?*

A. The best way to handle this situation is to probe by asking, "Can you tell me what you mean by that?" or, "Please tell me more about that." In any case, write down exactly what the responses are, regardless of your concerns.

Q. *Should I give encouragement and support during the interview process, such as, "That's right"?*

A. No. Your purpose is to be as objective as possible in asking the interview questions. Do not influence responses or shift the focus of the interview to one where the respondent is trying to please the interviewer. Likewise, do not interrupt the interview by explaining any answers that are "wrong" or appear off base. It is acceptable to say "Okay" in a neutral fashion after an answer is given.

In addition, if a respondent asks you if his answer to a question or interpretation to a page is right or wrong, you might respond with: "We're really just interested in your opinion, what makes sense to you."

Record *all* responses as given. There is no right or wrong when you're trying to identify potential problems.

Q. *How can I help the respondent feel comfortable?*

A. The best way is to have a friendly demeanor and be an active listener. This includes eye contact with your respondent, smiling when appropriate, assuming an open physical posture, and responding to comments with nonleading probes. Everyone likes to be asked their opinions about a topic with which they're familiar.

Experience Speaks . . . Advice on Interviewing Techniques from Several Experienced Interviewers for Learner Verification and Revision[1]

SELECTING TESTERS

- If possible, use testers from the same ethnic group.
- For foreign testers, make sure they don't change the questions or leave out questions that they don't care to ask.
- It is helpful if the testers have some counseling background.
- Consider two people to do interviews: one to ask questions and one to take notes.

INTRODUCTION OF THE INTERVIEW

- Consider saying: "We're asking lots of people about this booklet and trying to get an idea how *most* of them feel about it. It's in rough draft form here, so it's still easy to change it to make the finished one more clear."
- You may tell people during the introduction preamble that you didn't develop the piece. You're just checking it out, so you won't be offended by whatever they say.

READING OF THE MATERIAL

- When people are busy reading, the tester should be busy with some other activity nearby. It makes people nervous if you hover over them as you read.

DURING THE INTERVIEW

- Sometimes it's hard to get all the things written down that are being said. Some people want to say more and talk about the material. To solve this problem, write key words and phrases.
- Most people aren't prepared to offer ideas for changes/improvements. Stimulating examples or questions are needed to bring out their ideas.

AFTERWARD

- If possible, give the respondents a copy of the preliminary piece being tested and thank them. It makes them feel good about what they have done.

Sample Questionnaire for Interviewers to Evaluate Their Experience

Purpose: to give sponsor feedback on Learner Verification and Revision experience[2]

Would you help us by sharing your learner verification experience? We would like to know what you encountered and what we might be able to do in the future to make the process even more productive.

1. Total number of learner verification interviews conducted:
2. Total number of people approached who refused to participate:
3. Reasons given for refusal, if available:
4. Approximate minutes per interview:
5. What might we have included in the instructions that would have made the interviews more productive?
6. Is there anything that we could have left out?
7. What kind of problems did you encounter, if any?
8. We would like to have your opinion of the material itself. What do you think of it? Any suggestions for change?

Tabulation of Responses for Large Samples

For large samples (30 or more): A more formal spreadsheet tabulation is preferable for larger samples. Computer programs for spreadsheets offer several flexible frameworks for the layout. Using these tabular frameworks, it is easy to keyboard in the response data. A computer printout of the responses can provide you with an easy-to-scan tabulation so you can quickly identify trouble spots in the material being tested. An example of a computer-generated tabulation sheet is shown in Figure D-1. The figure shows only a part of the actual tabulation.

Function of questions: comprehension   acceptability

	Code	10. What is new?	11. First thing Jackie did to start?	12.a. Would you talk to your MD:	12b. If no, why?
		B1	B1	C	C
	03-10-16	It says she's walking and eating better.	Her clothes were too tight and her feet hurt (I asked the question again.) Oh, she talked to her doctor first.	No	Cause most of the time they give you a bunch of stuff to read and tell you not to eat so much and want you to starve yourself.
	03-10-17	She walks, she eats more fruits and vegetables.	She talked to her doctor about plan to lose weight.	Probably after I tried a diet.	Probably be cheaper.
	03-10-18	She's eating more fruits, vegs, and less fat.	She started eating less.	Yes	
	03-10-19	Eating more fruits and vegetables and less fat. out a simple plan.	Talk to her doctor, decided how much weight she wanted to lose and worked	Yes	
	03-10-20	Walk more.	She talked to her doctor.	I might if I had one.	
	03-10-21	She is walking, eating more fruits and vegetables	Talked to her doctor.	Yes	

Questions ▶

Code for respondents

Responses

FIGURE D-1

Tabulation of six responses to a booklet, "Jackie and Rhonda," for African Americans on losing weight and eating more fruits and vegetables to cut their risk of cancer. (*Source:* National Cancer Institute, Branch of Special Populations)

References

1. Feedback at National Cancer Institute conference (October 25, 1991): Barbara Pryor, RD, Columbus, OH; Sarah Furnas, RN, Philadelphia, PA; Joan Rupp, RD, San Diego, CA.
2. National Cancer Institute (1992): Branch of Special Populations, Nutrition Guideline for Ethnic Groups.

Index

207